FOODBORNE AND WATERBORNE DISEASES

THEIR EPIDEMIOLOGIC CHARACTERISTICS

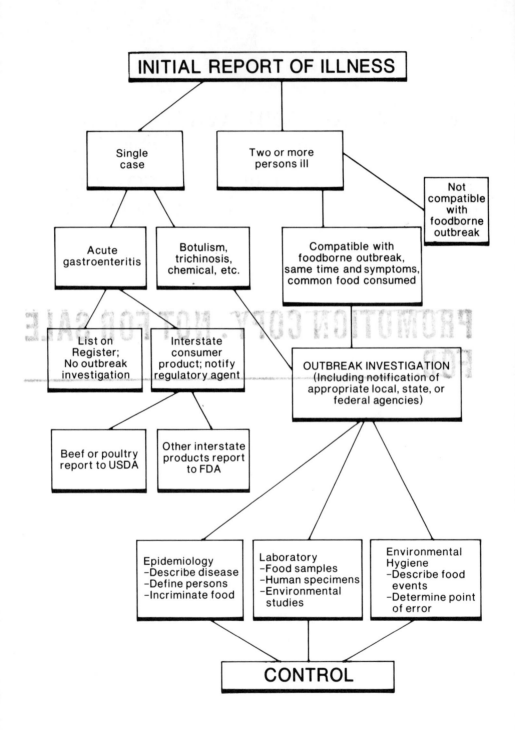

INITIAL REPORT OF ILLNESS

Single case

Two or more persons ill

Not compatible with foodborne outbreak

Acute gastroenteritis

Botulism, trichinosis, chemical, etc.

Compatible with foodborne outbreak, same time and symptoms, common food consumed

List on Register; No outbreak investigation

Interstate consumer product; notify regulatory agent

OUTBREAK INVESTIGATION (Including notification of appropriate local, state, or federal agencies)

Beef or poultry report to USDA

Other interstate products report to FDA

Epidemiology
–Describe disease
–Define persons
–Incriminate food

Laboratory
–Food samples
–Human specimens
–Environmental studies

Environmental Hygiene
–Describe food events
–Determine point of error

CONTROL

FOODBORNE AND WATERBORNE DISEASES

THEIR EPIDEMIOLOGIC CHARACTERISTICS

I. Jackson Tartakow, M.D., M.P.H.

Former Deputy Commissioner and
Epidemiologist
Department of Health
Nassau County, New York

John H. Vorperian, B.S.

Principal Sanitarian
Former Director
Bureau of Food and Beverage Control
Department of Health
Nassau County, New York

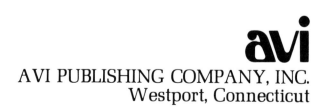

AVI PUBLISHING COMPANY, INC.
Westport, Connecticut

©Copyright 1981 by
THE AVI PUBLISHING COMPANY, INC.
Westport, Connecticut

Frontispiece Courtesy of Center for Disease Control, Atlanta

Library of Congress Cataloging in Publication Data

Tartakow, I   Jackson.
   Foodborne and waterborne diseases.

   Includes bibliographical references and index.
   1. Food poisoning. 2. Waterborne infection.
3. Epidemiology. I. Vorperian, John H., joint author.
II. Title. [DNLM: 1. Food poisoning. 2. Water
pollution. 3. Disease outbreaks—Prevention and
control. WC 268 T193f]
RA601.T34   614.4   80–24871
ISBN 0–87055–368–2

Printed in the United States of America by Eastern Graphics

Preface

The aim of this book is to familiarize the reader with certain characteristics of foodborne and waterborne diseases, a knowledge of which is necessary for their prevention and control.

The various infective and toxic agents—bacterial, viral, protozoan, parasitic, fungal, and chemical—capable of causing gastrointestinal disease or poisoning when ingested in contaminated food or water are discussed. Their incubation periods, their modes of transmission, and their periods of infectibility are presented. Their clinical signs and symptoms and laboratory diagnosis are outlined for their identification. Measures for their prevention are recommended.

Guidelines for the investigation and control of cases and of outbreaks of foodborne and waterborne diseases are given and examples of such investigations made by the senior author (I.J.T.) are presented as illustrations. Illness resulting from the mishandling of foods in food-processing, food-serving establishments and in the home is discussed. A summary of the reports prepared by the United States Public Health Service of the annual incidence of outbreaks of foodborne and waterborne diseases in the United States is also included.

A chapter is devoted to the discussion of plants that are poisonous when ingested. Another chapter describes poisons that are naturally contained in certain foods and types of illness they may cause.

References from many sources have been included. The reader will note that with the creation of the new Department of Education and its removal from the Department of Health, Education and Welfare (HEW) in 1980, the latter agency is now known as the Department of Health and Human Services (HHS).

As the use of technical and medical terminology could not be avoided, a glossary of any such terms that appear in the text is included.

Not only will the book prove instructive to students of schools of public health, administrative medicine, food sciences, hotel management, and those attending agricultural colleges, but also the material in the book should prove of assistance and guidance to health officers and personnel on their staff, such as epidemiologists, sanitary engineers, sanitarians, veterinarians, nurses, nutritionists, health educators, and social workers. Personnel in charge of quality control in food manufacturing plants may also benefit from the book.

It is hoped that it will provide valuable information to alert persons engaged in the various phases of the food industry whose responsibilities include providing the public with nourishment that is wholesome and free of pollution, contamination, and adulteration.

Officials concerned with maintaining the purity of drinking water will find essential facts for the prevention of contamination of the water supply in their charge.

Lastly, it is hoped that the reader will enjoy the occasional departure from pedantry, such as the philosophic discussion of sanitation, food, and water (Chapter 1), the occasional description of a historic epidemiologic occurrence such as "The Case of the Broad Street Pump" (Chapter 1), the relating of an interesting anecdote as "*Salmonella* vs Sanella" (Chapter 2), using a quotation from the past as Moses Maimonides on food poisoning (Chapter 5), as well as the descriptions of some of the experiences of the senior author in the performance of his duties as epidemiologist in a county with a population of approximately 1,750,000 people.

I. JACKSON TARTAKOW
JOHN H. VORPERIAN

October 1, 1980

Dedicated to our esteemed colleague, Dr. George G. Cook, who for many years served as Chairman of the Food Technology Department at SUNY, Farmingdale, N.Y.

Contents

1

Introduction

A microscopic layer of fecal organisms may be said to cover the whole of humanity, the thickness varying directly with the degree of personal hygiene of each individual and the type of sanitation existing in the environment of the locality he inhabits. This view may be confirmed by the ubiquity of *Escherichia coli* outside of its natural habitat, the colon. In spite of this condition, these organisms, except for some unusual pathogenic strains, do not produce disease. One person, however, may transmit an intestinal disease to another if he himself has or has had the disease and has become an acute, temporary, convalescent, or chronic carrier with his feces containing the causative microorganism.

Such a carrier, if he is engaged in the production, preparation, or service of foods consumed by persons outside his own household, constitutes a danger to the community. He must therefore be prevented from engaging in his occupation until he is fully recovered and it is established by laboratory examination that he has been relieved of his carrier state.

All food handlers must adhere to strict sanitary techniques so as not to endanger the public health. One of the simplest and most effective measures they must observe before handling any food is the washing of hands, particularly after the use of the toilet. Another is the prompt storage of all raw and prepared foods under proper refrigeration (below 7.2°C or 45°F) so as to arrest the multiplication of any pathogen that may have been introduced into the food.

In addition to the spread of foodborne diseases by man, a number of domestic and game animals may also be carriers of organisms capable of causing enteric diseases in humans. This is especially true of animals whose flesh is eaten by man. For example: turkeys and other fowl may transmit salmonellosis to man; pork, beef and fish, if harboring various types of tapeworms, may transmit them if improperly cooked; pork is also capable of causing trichinosis; tularemia may be acquired by the ingestion of inadequately cooked meat of infected wild rabbits; and raw

1

milk from infected cows will cause brucellosis. Fortunately, the high temperatures required for cooking such meats and the pasteurization of milk inactivate the pathogens and protect man from infection. Even contact with the urine or feces of the family dog or other pets (turtles) may result in illness by hand-to-mouth spread or contamination of food.

When such tainted food is eaten, the invading organisms on entering the gastrointestinal tract multiply in large numbers and cause various forms of gastroenteritis. The infective agents may be bacteria, viruses, helminths (worms), or protozoa. Among the diseases caused by bacteria are salmonellosis and typhoid fever, shigellosis, cholera, streptococcal sore throat, and food poisoning by *Clostridium botulinum* and *Staphylococcus aureus*. The latter two produce an enterotoxin in the contaminated food before it is ingested, and it is the toxin rather than the bacilli in the digestive system that produces the illness.

Viral contamination of food may result in viral hepatitis if the food is carelessly handled by a person suffering or convalescing from the disease and harboring the virus in his feces. Other foodborne viral diseases are lymphocytic choriomeningitis and epidemic hemorrhagic fever which infected United States troops in Korea.

Worms, among them intestinal roundworms, tapeworms, and flukes (nematodes), may be transmitted to man by infected persons or animals. The eggs or larvae are introduced into salads or other foods either by hands contaminated with human or animal feces, or by soil containing the eggs. In the intestinal tract, the eggs hatch and migrate to other organs by way of the lymphatic or circulatory system.

Protozoan foodborne infections may also be transmitted by fecal contamination of food or water; amebiasis (amebic dysentery) and giardiasis are two such diseases.

The question may arise as to how one can tell that an item of food is spoiled and unfit for consumption (the term ordinarily used is "human consumption," but that is avoided since any food unfit for human consumption is also unfit for animal consumption). Most meats, including fowl, fish, and shrimp, usually have a disagreeable odor when they are spoiled or contaminated. In addition, uncooked fish meat that pulls away easily from bones; dressed fowl that is sticky to the touch; and beef, pork, and similar fresh meats that have become slimy should be considered unusable as food.

A good test for canned foods is to note their tops and bottoms to determine whether they have swelled out into dome-like shapes. This indicates that the contents have spoiled, usually because of a slightly open seam permitting a gas-producing microorganism to enter and contaminate the contents. If an attempt is made to open the can, there will be a rush of escaping gas and an abnormal odor will ensue.

Salads such as those made from chicken, eggs, tuna, or ham must be kept refrigerated at a temperature below 7.2°C (45°F) until ready to eat. Similarly, custard-filled pastries and cold cuts require constant refrigeration to arrest the growth of any pathogenic organisms that they may contain.

Food is not the only vehicle of transmission of gastrointestinal diseases. Water polluted either directly with feces from patients or carriers or indirectly by fecal containing sewage is another form of spread. Epidemics of typhoid fever and cholera in the past have incriminated polluted water supplies.

Attention is called to a particular phase pertaining to water that may surprise many people. Few persons realize that the water they drink, cook with, and bathe in has been *recycled* as is done with old newspapers and discarded aluminum. The glass of crystal clear refreshing water one is drinking may contain many molecules of water that have passed one or more times through the digestive and urinary tracts of several other humans. The urine and other fluids that are excreted by living beings consist of water in which body waste products are dissolved. These undergo some form of sewage treatment and their diluent (water) is then returned as an effluent to the surface, joining a body of water such as a stream or lake that may serve as a water source. Should the effluent empty into the sea, the molecules of water under discussion may be returned to the atmosphere by evaporation and be condensed as rain or snow falling to the ground.

In rural areas, the liquid contents of cesspools percolate through the sandy soil that acts as nature's filter, oxidizing its organic matter and straining out the bacteria that it may contain. The filtrate thus reaches an underground impervious stratum or water table and may be tapped when a well is sunk, or it may appear on the surface as a spring.

Molecules of water thus reconditioned by nature may pass through a number of persons. They do not cause disease *per se* unless they are recontaminated with pathogenic organisms shed by sick persons or carriers or are polluted by a toxic chemical waste product.

An early classic illustration that disease may be conveyed by water was made in Great Britain in 1854 by John Snow, epidemiologist, and John York, Secretary and Surveyor of the Cholera Inquiry Committee (Snow and York 1855). The study is known as "The Case of the Broad Street Pump." Cholera at that time was prevalent in London but occurred with epidemic intensity and great fatality in the district about Broad Street. Epidemiologic study of the epidemic revealed that most of the victims had used water from the well located on that street. On examination of the well, it was found that the mortar joints between the bricks making up its sides had been washed away and served as a sieve through which

drainage from an adjoining similarly defective cesspool had been perco-
lating for a considerable period of time. The cesspool served a house in
which there were 4 severe cases of cholera. The epidemic was promptly
arrested by a simple procedure, namely, the removal of the handle of the
Broad Street pump.

A markedly significant reduction in the incidence of foodborne and
waterborne diseases has been brought about by improved living conditions, modern sanitation, chlorination of water supplies, pasteurization
of milk, prophylactic immunization of contacts and susceptibles, introduction of mechanical refrigeration, sanitary design of food equipment,
and prompt treatment of infected persons. Typhoid fever may be cited
as an example. Sir William Osler, the renowned physician, has stated
that "typhoid fever has been one of the great scourges of armies and has
killed and maimed more than powder and shot." He pointed out that in
the Spanish American War in the national encampments among 107,773
men, there were 20,738 cases of typhoid fever with 1580 deaths. Camp
pollution, contamination of the water supply, and fly transmission to
food were blamed for the outbreaks. On the other hand, in World War I,
with the application of modern sanitation and the vaccination of all
enlisted men, typhoid fever did not prevail to any extent.

Public health laws pertaining to food manufacturing, processing and
handling, periodic inspection of establishments where food is prepared
and served, and the education through various media of commercial food
handlers, as well as housewives, in the proper preparation and storage of
foods have done much in the control and prevention of foodborne diseases.

Modern indoor plumbing with the sanitary disposal of feces, proper
sewage treatment, and the protection, purification, and chlorination of
public water supplies may be said to be responsible for the rare occurrence of waterborne outbreaks.

In general, it may be said that with few exceptions man serves as the
main reservoir of infection of the more serious gastrointestinal diseases.
When he is infected, his feces contain the organisms that are responsible
for his illness and capable of causing the disease in others. It is therefore
of the utmost importance for those of us who are charged with the
preservation of the public health to exercise every effort to prevent one
man's feces, no matter how infinitesimal the quantity may be, from
entering another man's gastrointestinal tract through the foods he eats
and the liquids he drinks.

In discussing the numerous diseases transmitted by food and water, a
certain degree of repetition is unavoidable. A high percentage of the
diseases have similar signs and symptoms with the majority of them
having, among other complaints, the gastrointestinal triad: vomiting,

abdominal cramps, and diarrhea. There may also be similarity in their mode of transmission, in their method of control, and in the steps necessary for their prevention. Rather than referring the reader to previous chapters in the book, pertinent information for each disease is described even if it has already been mentioned in relation to another disease.

REFERENCES

GELDREICH, E.E. and BORDNER, R.H. 1971. Fecal contamination of fruits and vegetables during cultivation and processing for market. A review. J. Milk Food Technol. *34*, 184.

HELDERMAN, D.R. 1974. Factors influencing air-borne contamination of foods. A review. J. Food Sci. *39*, 922.

McBRIDE, M.E., DUNCAN, W.C. and KNOX, J.M. 1977. The environment and the microbial ecology of human skin. Appl. Environ. Microbiol. *33*, 603.

NOBLE, W.C. 1975. Dispersal of skin microorganisms. Br. J. Dermatol. *93*, 477.

SMITH, H. 1977. Microbial surfaces in relation to pathogenicity. Bacteriol. Rev. *41*, 475.

SNOW, J. and YORK, J. 1855. Report on the Cholera Outbreak in the Parish of James, Westminster, July 1855. J. Churchill, London.

2

Salmonellosis

Before we turn our attention to the microorganism known as *Salmonella*, it is interesting to note that a discussion regarding the bacillus, usually reserved for persons of a scientific background, recently took place among the members of the United States Senate. It was not the pathogenicity of the organism or the potential danger that it presented to their constituents that concerned the legislators. It was merely a question of semantics and its alleged influence on one particular industry.

According to an editorial that appeared in *Nutrition Today* in 1967 (Enloe 1967), Senator Warren G. Magnuson of the state of Washington introduced in June of that year a bill (S-2019) that would alter, for the first time in the history of the United States Congress, the name of a microorganism and of the disease that it causes. The senator's contribution to medical nomenclature stated:

Be it enacted by the Senate and House of Representatives of the United States of America in Congress assembled, that (a) it is the policy of the Federal Government that the term "sanella" should be employed to designate the particular genus of bacteria presently designated by the term "salmonella" and that the term "sanellosis" shall be employed to designate the particular disease presently designated by the term "salmonellosis."

The bill then went on to command that all "departments, agencies and instrumentalities of the Federal Government . . . shall comply with the policy . . . ."

It is suspected that this exceptional piece of legislature was proposed in response to pressure brought by the salmon industry lobby that feels that the American public erroneously associates the bacterium *Salmonella* with their favorite product, and that there is a causative relationship between the fish and the disease salmonellosis.

It is purely coincidental that the name of the scientist who first described the *Salmonella* bacillus, and after whom it was named, should

6

be synonymous with that of the anadromous fish that breeds in the rivers in the senator's state. The only time an actual association would be established between the bacillus and the fish would be if the two were to come together because of faulty processing or handling. The public might then see a front-page news headline such as "Salmon Causes Salmonellosis."

To our knowledge the senator's bill has not become a law and it is still legal to refer to the organism and the disease by their traditional names. These shall be used throughout the discussion that follows.

Characteristics

Salmonellosis, formerly referred to as paratyphoid infection, is an acute form of enteritis caused by a Gram-negative rod-shaped bacillus known as *Salmonella*, named after Dr. D.E. Salmon, who first described it in 1885. There are more than 1000 different strains or serotypes of the organism with additional ones being constantly uncovered. The various strains are differentiated by agglutination tests. Some strains have greater pathogenicity than others with many capable of attacking animals as well as man. The types most commonly found in the United States are *S. typhimurium, S. enteritidis, S. heidelberg, S. paratyphi A* and *B, S. infantum, S. choleraesuis, S. newport, S. st. paul, S. derby,* and *S. oranienburg.* The most pathogenic member is *S. typhi,* which causes typhoid fever and is discussed at length in Chapter 3.

Although cases occur throughout the year, the greatest number is usually reported between the months of July and September (see Fig. 2.2).

Salmonellosis is usually a form of gastroenteritis characterized by a sudden onset with fever, griping and severe abdominal pain, nausea and vomiting, anorexia (lack of appetite), foul smelling diarrhea, weakness, and dehydration. Although *Salmonella* usually invades and localizes itself in the gastrointestinal system, in extreme instances it may invade other systems (such as respiratory, central nervous, genitourinary, or cardiovascular) causing pneumonia, meningitis, pyelonephritis, endocarditis, and pericarditis. Severity depends on the serotype of the invading organism, the dosage of bacteria ingested, and certain host factors such as age, debilitation, and concurrent illness. The fatality rate is about 4%, the very young and very old being most vulnerable.

The incubation period of salmonellosis or the time required for symptoms to appear after ingestion is 6 to 48 hr, but illness usually occurs in 12 to 24 hr and may last from 3 days to 3 weeks during which time the patient may be a temporary or convalescent carrier excreting *Salmonella*

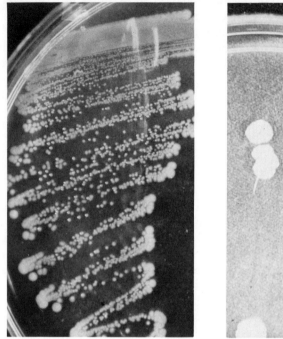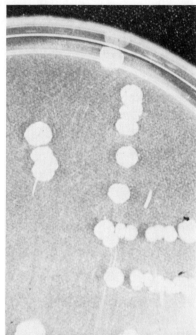

Courtesy of Elliot Scientific Corp. and Abbott Laboratories

FIG. 2.1. *SALMONELLA* SPECIES
LEFT—Culture on Endo agar: colorless, non–lactose fermenting colonies.
RIGHT—Pure culture on Endo agar.

in his feces and capable of contaminating food consumed by other persons.

Sources of Infection

Although man serves as the main reservoir of infection, animals, especially those whose flesh serves as food, such as turkeys and chickens, or those present in the home as dogs and pet turtles, also play a role in the spread of salmonellosis.

As previously stated, salmonellosis is transmitted by the ingestion of the causative organisms in food contaminated by infected feces from man or animal. Among foods most frequently involved because of their ability to support the growth and multiplication of *Salmonella* are whole eggs and egg products (frozen or dried eggs, egg albumin, and egg yolk, especially from duck eggs), poultry, meat and meat products, commer-

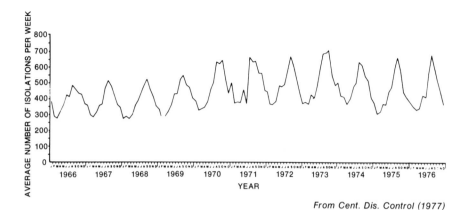

From Cent. Dis. Control (1977)

FIG. 2.2. THE REPORTED NUMBER OF ISOLATIONS OF SALMONELLAE FROM HU-
MANS, BY MONTH, UNITED STATES, 1966–1976

cially processed meats and poultry, pies, sausages, products containing
eggs, unpasteurized whole milk, and powdered milk and milk products.

The responsibility for the transmission of salmonellosis to man by
domestic animals rests on the shoulders of man, as he infects the animals
he raises or breeds with the feed he offers them. Animal feed and mixes
often are made from waste animal by-products such as fish meal, poultry meal, meat scraps, and tankage—mostly the refuse of animals. These
products are primary sources of *Salmonella*. As they are intended for
animal use, they are processed with little regard for cleanliness and
sanitation. The feed, frequently contaminated, infects the animal that
eats it. The animal is eventually slaughtered for human consumption and
its intestinal contents or diseased tissues contaminate his flesh, thus
infecting man if the meat is inadequately stored or improperly cooked.

Even the innocuous pet turtle may become a carrier and cause human
salmonellosis, particularly in young children. The turtle becomes infected, like other animals, by being given contaminated feed. Children invariably handle the pets and contaminate their hands with fecal containing
tank water. They then fail to wash their hands before eating, thus
infecting themselves. Cultures of patients' feces and of tank water have
revealed the presence of the same serotype of salmonella on numerous
occasions.

Sometimes illness has been blamed on canned foods. Such views are
unfounded as the organisms are not found in unopened cans since the
processing timing and temperatures of canning preclude the survival of
any microorganism. Contamination of such foods takes place after the
can has been opened and its contents handled in an unsanitary manner

by a carrier with soiled hands or by utensils. However, one must avoid dented and swollen cans as their contents invariably are contaminated perhaps through an opening in the seam following a fall.

Prevention

The prevention of salmonellosis may be accomplished by observing the following recommendations:

(1) All foodstuffs from animal sources should be thoroughly cooked.
(2) Avoid recontamination of foods after cooking by careful handling.
(3) Avoid eating raw, dirty, or cracked eggs.
(4) Pasteurize milk and milk products.
(5) Refrigerate prepared foods as well as leftovers during storage before use.
(6) Educate food handlers and homemakers in the importance of adequate refrigeration of foods, handwashing before food preparation, maintaining a sanitary kitchen, and protecting foods from rodent and insect contamination.
(7) Periodic meat and poultry inspection by trained personnel with supervision of abattoirs, as well as federal inspection of animals (cattle, sheep, goats, swine, and horses) in interstate shipment with the purpose of excluding diseased animals and to control the sanitary handling of meats.
(8) Animal feed should be cooked or heat treated against contamination with *Salmonella*.
(9) Protect foods from contamination with rat or mouse feces and from contact with houseflies.

Diagnosis and Treatment

Laboratory diagnosis of salmonellosis is most satisfactory when *Salmonella* are isolated from both the suspected food (if available) and the patient's feces. It appears in the feces during the acute symptoms and often disappears when the symptoms subside. Agglutination tests are not significant as the titer is not sufficiently increased to be diagnostic.

The following steps may be followed for the care of patients:

(1) All cases and outbreaks must be reported to local health authorities.
(2) Infected person's feces and soiled articles should be disinfected; if home has modern flush toilet connected to an adequate sewage treatment system, patient's feces may be discharged untreated directly into toilet.

(3) Fecal specimens should be obtained for laboratory examination from family contacts to determine whether any of them are mild undiagnosed cases or carriers.

(4) Treatment of the patient is symptomatic and supportive; with the exception of chloramphenicol, the antibiotics fail to shorten the period of illness; they tend to prolong the carrier state and may lead to resistant strains.

(5) Infected persons must be excluded from the handling of food or caring of children or the elderly until fecal cultures are free of *Salmonella* for 3 consecutive days.

Commercial Importance and Public Health

In recent years salmonellosis has assumed considerable commercial importance. The discovery of dried milk invaded with *Salmonella* that resulted in a recall of several nationally distributed products may be cited as a case in point. The occurrence of an outbreak traced to a producer or processor or to a restaurant, if publicized by any of the news media, will result in loss of public confidence and will invariably have a deleterious effect on its future.

It would be to the economic advantage to the processor, distributor, and food-service establishment owner to control the incidence of food-borne disease by instituting sanitary control measures through self-inspection in addition to complying with plant regulations and recommendations pertaining to sanitation. They should remember that good sanitation is good business. When an item of food, regardless of its cost, is of questionable quality, restaurateurs should heed the slogan, "When in doubt, throw it out!"

Salmonellosis may occur in a single individual or in an outbreak involving a number of persons who have partaken of a common contaminated item of food at a restaurant, banquet, or gathering. The food may have been contaminated at its source or during its preparation. Such outbreaks are often reported by hospitals, nursing homes for the aged, and institutions for the care of children.

Contaminated water as well as food may be responsible for the spread of salmonellosis. A severe epidemic of *S. typhimurium* diarrhea involving more than 15,000 cases occurred in Riverside, California, in 1965. It was due to the contamination of the unchlorinated deep water supply.

In order to demonstrate how outbreaks of that nature are epidemiologically investigated to determine their source and control further spread, a report of such an investigation follows in its entirety.

INVESTIGATION OF OUTBREAK OF *SALMONELLA* ENTERITIS IN BALDWIN, N.Y.

An outbreak of enteritis occurred among the members and guests of the Baldwin Chapter of the Order of the Eastern Star following a meeting on the evening of Feb. 15.

The attention of the Department of Health was called to the outbreak by Dr. O.A.D., who on Feb. 17 phoned and reported 5 patients with severe enteritis who stated that they had attended the Eastern Star meeting and partaken of some collations served after the meeting. An investigation was begun on the following morning.

Scope of Investigation

The study included the following:

(1) Obtainment of clinical and epidemiologic histories from as great a number of guests as possible in order to determine the nature of illness.
(2) Collection of data regarding the distribution of cases among members of the Order and their guests.
(3) Determination of the articles of food consumed by affected as well as unaffected persons.
(4) Survey of conditions under which the foods were prepared, stored, and served to the members and guests.
(5) Determination of the infective agent and its mode of transmission through submission and examination of stool specimens and food samples.
(6) Discovery of the source of infection.

Investigation

By interviewing the 5 reported cases, the names of other persons known by them to be ill, as well as the names of the officers of the Order, were obtained. Clinical and epidemiologic histories were thus personally secured from 29 patients and stool specimens requested from 21 of them. A conference was held with the matron and secretary of the Order and a list of the members was obtained from them. The list contained 104 names, but that was not considered the total number of persons exposed as the new matron had been installed at the meeting and several members had brought guests for the occasion.

As it appeared a difficult task for the investigator to see all the persons involved within a limited period of time, a letter and questionnaire were sent to each of the 104 members. The letter was as follows:

Dear Madam:

Your name appears on the list of guests who attended a meeting of the Baldwin Chapter Order of Eastern Star at the Masonic Temple in Baldwin on the evening of February 15. This department has been informed that collations were served that evening and that a number of guests became ill shortly thereafter.

As you know, one of the functions of the Health Department is to investigate and whenever possible to determine the cause of reported outbreaks of disease. To make certain that the true nature and extent of this outbreak are determined exactly, we request that you complete promptly and fully the enclosed forms, one for each member of your family in attendance at the meeting, and mail same in the enclosed self-addressed stamped envelope.

Your full cooperation may be of considerable assistance to us in our efforts to prevent a similar occurrence in the future.

> Sincerely yours,
> I.J. Tartakow, M.D.
> Epidemiologist

One or more of the following questionnaires and a self-addressed stamped envelope were enclosed with the letter:

NAME _____ AGE_____ SEX_____
ADDRESS_____   _____
         (Street & Number)   (Village or City)

Please indicate which of the following items of food were eaten by you at the February 15 meeting at Masonic Temple, Baldwin:

        Turkey Salad   Yes_____   No_____
        Cake   Yes_____   No_____
        Coffee   Yes_____   No_____

Did you become ill following the dinner? Yes _____ No _____

If so, at what time_____p.m. or a.m. Date_____

Which of the following symptoms did you have? (Please check)

        Chill _____   Nausea _____
        Fever _____   Vomiting _____
        Headache _____   Abdominal cramps __
        Sweat _____   Diarrhea _____

How long did the illness last? _____hours _____days

Were you attended by a physician? _____ If so, indicate:

    1. Name of physician _____
    2. Address _____
    3. Date of visit _____

If known, list guests other than members you brought to the meeting.

    1. _____
    2. _____
    3. _____
    4. _____
    5. _____
    6. _____

If information was secured from individual other than the person named at **the** top of sheet, give name of informant: _____

Name of investigator_____

It was thus possible to obtain from the questionnaires completed **by** these members the additional names of 46 guests. Questionnaires **were** sent to a total of 150 persons. Completed questionnaires were **returned** by 118 of them, or 78.7%. Analysis of the data so obtained revealed **the** information given below.

Number of Cases

There was a total of 91 persons attacked out of the 118 who **submitted** information, making an incidence rate of 77.1%. Females numbered **88** and males 30, the attack rates being nearly identical for both **sexes** (females 77.3%; males 76.7%) (Table 2.1).

TABLE 2.1. ATTACK RATES BY SEX DISTRIBUTION

	Total	Attacked Number	%	Not Attacked Number	%
Females	88	68	77.3	20	22.7
Males	30	23	76.7	7	23.3
Total	118	91	77.1	27	23.0

Clinical Character of Cases

In general, the clinical manifestations of the cases were similar. Diarrhea with from 2 to 12 watery and in some instances bloody stools **per** day during illness occurred in 92.3% of the cases and was accompanied **by** abdominal cramps of varied degree in 79.1%. Fever was reported **in** 75.8% and chills in 73.6%. Nausea occurred in 67.0% and vomiting **in** 61.5%. Complaints of headache were made by 52.7% and sweats **by** 49.5% (Table 2.2).

TABLE 2.2. FREQUENCY OF SYMPTOMS OF 91 CASES OF ENTERITIS

Symptom	Cases Number	%
Diarrhea	84	92.3
Cramps	72	79.1
Fever	69	75.8
Chills	67	73.6
Nausea	61	67.0
Vomiting	56	61.5
Headache	48	52.7
Sweats	45	49.5

The average duration of illness was 7.2 days. Three patients recovered within 24 hr and 1 was ill for 1 month. Illness was sufficiently severe in 68 instances for patients to seek medical consultation. As far as is known, all recovered completely except for weakness. There was no fatality.

Incubation Period of Outbreak

The business portion of the meeting terminated at about 10:00 P.M., and collations were served between 10:30 and 11:00 P.M. Over 80% of the patients became ill within 24 hr of the repast. The earliest case occurred in about 2 hr and the last case 80 hr later. The mean incubation period or interval between the eating of the food and the beginning of illness was found to be 18.2 hr (Table 2.3).

TABLE 2.3.   INTERVAL BETWEEN EATING OF TURKEY SALAD AND ONSET OF SYMP-TOMS

Hours from Infection (X)	Number of Cases (F)	(FX)
2	1	2
3	1	3
4	2	8
5	2	10
6	1	6
7	2	14
8	14	112
9	1	9
10	2	20
11	2	22
12	4	48
13	3	39
14	2	28
15	3	45
16	8	124
17	6	102
18	9	162
19	1	19
20	5	100
21	1	21
22	2	44
23	1	23
24	2	48
27	1	27
28	1	28
31	1	31
35	2	70
36	4	144
40	2	80
42	2	84
48	1	48
55	1	55
80	1	80
Total	91 (N)	1656 (ΣFX)

$$\text{Mean} = \frac{\Sigma FX}{N} = \frac{1656}{91} = 18.2 \text{ hr}$$

Possible Factors of Causation

The explosive nature of the outbreak, the clinical character, and the selective distribution of the cases considered together suggested strongly that food was the most logical medium of conveyance of the causative agent. Contagion or personal contact between cases could be precluded as a factor on the same basis. Water may be ruled out as the probable vehicle of transmission since the Masonic Temple where the meeting was held is served by a public water supply.

The collation served the evening of the meeting consisted of (1) turkey salad, (2) sponge cake with jelly layer and icing, and (3) coffee with half cream and half milk ("Half & Half," Evans-Amityville Dairy).

Tabulation of the information on the 118 questionnaires disclosed that of the 91 persons who became ill, 100% ate turkey salad, 74.8% ate cake, and 70.3% drank coffee. Of the 27 persons who remained well, only 44.4% ate turkey salad, 63.0% ate cake, and 70.4% drank coffee (Table 2.4).

TABLE 2.4. NUMBER AND PERCENTAGE OF ATTACKED AND UNATTACKED PERSONS WHO ATE VARIOUS FOODS

| | Guests Who Ate Various Foods | | | |
| | Attacked | | Not Attacked | |
Food	Number	%	Number	%
Turkey salad	91	100.0	12	44.4
Cake	68	74.8	17	63.0
Coffee	64	70.3	19	70.4

It is evident from Table 2.4 that turkey salad was the only item of food eaten by every one of the attacked persons. The difference between the percentages of attacked and unattacked persons who ate turkey salad appears considerably greater than that between those who ate cake or drank coffee. It is felt that this difference is significant in incriminating the turkey salad. Out of a total of 103 guests who ate the salad, 91 of them or 88.4% became ill.

In 9 instances guests took portions of leftover salad home to be eaten by household members. In each of these situations the person who ate it became ill. This is additional evidence pointing to the turkey salad as the suspected food.

Mode of Contamination

With the turkey salad established epidemiologically as the most probable medium of conveyance of the causative agent of the outbreak, the question arose as to how it became contaminated.

Flies, roaches, mice, or other vermin may be ruled out as the sanitary and hygienic conditions of the kitchen where the salad was prepared appeared satisfactory.

Investigation of the preparation of the turkey salad revealed that a number of persons participated in it. Three frozen dressed turkeys weighing about 9 kg (20 lb) each were purchased from a chain meat market 3 days before the meeting. Three members were assigned a turkey apiece with instructions to cook it at home and deliver it to the Temple on the morning of the meeting.

One woman cooked her turkey 2 days before the meeting, cooled it for 3 hr, sliced the meat, and refrigerated it until it was time to transport it to the Temple.

Each of the other 2 women cooked their birds the evening before the meeting, left it all night on their porches, and sliced it on the morning of the meeting just before transporting it.

Preparation of the salad in the kitchen of the Temple was begun at 9:30 A.M. Six other women assisted in cutting up celery, lettuce, green peppers, and sliced pickles and in cubing the turkey meat. These ingredients were placed into 3 large aluminum kettles (12 and 15 qt sizes). Three of the women admitted that as no spoon or ladle was available for mixing the ingredients, they resorted to primitive means and used their hands for that purpose. Two of the kettles were then placed in the refrigerator at the Temple and as there was no room for the third pot, it was kept in a cement stairwell leading to the back yard.

At about 4 P.M. the matron brought in 4 qt jars of mayonnaise, took the pots out of the refrigerator, and added the mayonnaise. She also mixed the salad with her hands. The 3 pots were allegedly forced into the refrigerator where they remained until the salad was served on paper dishes between 10:30 and 11 P.M.

Examination of the refrigerator in question revealed it to be an old discarded model used only on special occasions—about twice a month— the rest of the time it was disconnected. It had been specially plugged in that morning but its efficiency and ability to attain a desirable temperature are questioned.

The storage of the salad in the large cylindrical kettles between the time of its preparation and serving is definitely unsatisfactory. Even in a modern efficient refrigerator it is doubtful whether the center of the mass of salad in each pot could have been sufficiently cooled to prevent bacterial growth.

On conferring with each of 7 members who participated in the preparation of the salad, none was found to have any injury or infection of the hands. Four of them ate some turkey salad and became ill. It was learned that the matron who added the mayonnaise and mixed the salad with her hands had had some abdominal cramps for about 4 hr previous to that activity and had had a loose bowel movement that afternoon. Her illness subsequently became quite severe and lasted 6 days. The assumption that the turkey salad was most probably contaminated by this person may therefore be made with some certainty.

Infective Agent

According to Dack (1956), the time intervals present between the eating of incriminated food and the beginning of gastrointestinal symptoms due to various specific agents have been found to be as follows: botulism, average 1 to 2 days; *Staphylococcus* enterotoxin, 1 to 6 hr, average 2½ to 3 hr; *Salmonella*, 7 to 72 hr, average 12 to 24 hr; *Streptococcus* (alpha type), 5 to 18 hr. McClung (1945), who described 4 outbreaks of food poisoning due to the enterotoxin of *Clostridium perfringens (C. welchii)* in freshly cooked chicken, found the incubation period to be from 8 to 12 hr after meals.

Botulism, *Staphylococcus* enterotoxin, mineral poisoning due to insecticides, rodenticides, or other chemicals, or poisonous plants such as mushrooms, could be eliminated as possible causative factors from the epidemiologic and clinical histories and incubation period.

The mean incubation period of 18.2 hr, the type of illness, and its average duration of 7.2 days point to infection with a bacterial agent that requires time for multiplication in the intestinal tract before infection is manifest. The most probable bacterial agent capable of meeting these conditions is *Salmonella*.

Laboratory Findings

Fortunately, it was possible to obtain samples of cake and turkey salad from one of the guests. She had taken some of each home for her husband who ate part of the salad and became ill. On culture of the specimens at the Division of Laboratories & Research, Nassau County Department of Health, a member of the *Salmonella* group was isolated from the salad. Upon further study, it was identified as *Salmonella reading* by both the National Salmonella Center in New York City and the New York State Department of Health. No enteric pathogen was isolated from the cake.

Examination of stool specimens submitted by 15 patients revealed the presence of a *Salmonella* organism of the same species. No dysentery or typhoid bacillus was found.

The stools of the 4 persons, including the matron who had helped prepare the salad and had become ill, were examined. *Salmonella reading* was isolated from feces submitted by the matron and one of the members (Table 2.5).

TABLE 2.5. MEMBERS WHO HELPED PREPARE TURKEY SALAD

Name	Ate Turkey Salad	Illness	Lab Exam	Report
R.F.[1]	Yes	Yes	Yes	*Salmonella reading*
L.H.	Yes	Yes	Yes	*Salmonella reading*
A.M.	No	No	No	None
E.B.	No	No	No	None
M.L.	Turkey meat only	No	No	None
E.G.	Yes	Yes	Yes	Negative
P.J.	Yes	Yes	Yes	Negative

[1]Matron.

In order to determine whether any of the infected persons became carriers of the *Salmonella* bacillus, the following letter was sent to each of the 37 physicians whose names were given in the questionnaires as having attended the 68 patients:

Dear Doctor:

It has been reported to this department that the above mentioned person(s) became ill with gastroenteritis following the eating of collation at a meeting of the Order of the Eastern Star, Baldwin Chapter, on February 15. Laboratory examination of stools of a number of involved guests and of samples of food served that evening revealed that illness was caused by *Salmonella reading.*

Because of the possibility that a carrier state for salmonella may develop in persons who had an acute infection, it is advisable to culture stools from such individuals even though symptoms have subsided.

As the above mentioned persons reported that you rendered treatment during illness, your help is requested in securing stool specimens for culture in order to determine whether the carrier state has resulted. Two specimens at least 24 hours apart are recommended.

Containers for the mailing of specimens to the Division of Laboratories & Research may be obtained at our main office at 1053 Franklin Avenue, Garden City, or at our supply substation at South Nassau Communities Hospital, Oceanside.

Your cooperation in preventing the spread of this infection would be appreciated.

Very truly yours,
I.J. Tartakow, M.D., Epidemiologist

A letter was also sent to those patients who had no medical attention inviting them to submit stools for the same purpose.

Summary and Conclusion

An outbreak of salmonellosis occurred among members and guests of the Baldwin Chapter of the Order of Eastern Star following a meeting on

February 15 at which collation was served. Out of 150 guests, epidemiologic information was obtained from 118. It was found that 91 of them became ill, giving an incidence rate of 77.1%.

The clinical manifestations of the cases were in general similar, with diarrhea, abdominal cramps, fever, and chills predominant. The mean incubation period was 18.2 hr. Illness lasted an average of 7.2 days and fortunately there was no fatality.

The epidemiologic evidence obtained during the study incriminated turkey salad prepared on the same morning, mixed with bare hands by 4 women, improperly stored in large deep pots, and inadequately refrigerated. One of the persons who mixed it had early symptoms of enteritis—abdominal cramps and diarrhea—for about 4 hr previously.

Salmonella reading was isolated from a sample of turkey salad, as well as from stool specimens from 15 patients, including the person who mixed the salad and had cramps and diarrhea previous to the meeting.

It appears reasonable to assume that this person was either a carrier of *Salmonella* or had an early case of *Salmonella* enteritis at that time, and when she mixed the salad with her hands contaminated it with the pathogen. Improper storage for about 5 hr fostered its multiplication and resulted in the outbreak.

It was recommended to the secretary of the Order that professional determination be made of the efficiency of the refrigerator at the Temple. The utilization of flat pans rather than deep pots for storage of food and proper utensils for its preparation in the future was advised.

REFERENCES

ASERKOFF, B., SCHROEDER, S.A. and BRACHMAN, P.S. 1970. Salmonellosis in the United States—A five-year review. Am. J. Epidemiol. *92*, 13.

BAINE, W.B., GANGAROSA, E.J., BENNETT, J.V. and BARKER, W.H., JR. 1973. Institutional salmonellosis. J. Infect. Dis. *128*, 357.

BARTLETT, K.H., TRUST, T.J. and LIOR, H. 1977. Small pet aquarium frogs as a source of *Salmonella*. Appl. Environ. Microbiol. *33*, 1026.

BERENSON, A.D. 1970. Control of Communicable Diseases in Man. American Public Health Association, Washington, D.C.

BLACK, P.H. *et al.* 1960. Salmonella—A review of some unusual aspects. N. Engl. J. Med. *262*, 811, 864, 921.

CENT. DIS. CONTROL. 1977A. Foodborne and Waterborne Disease Outbreaks. Annual Summary 1976. Center for Disease Control, Atlanta, Ga.

CENT. DIS. CONTROL. 1977B. *Salmonella* in pre-cooked beef. Morbidity Mortality *26*, 310.

CHERRY, W.B., DAVIS, B.R., EDWARDS, F.R. and HOGAN, R.B. 1954. A simple procedure for the identification of the genus *Salmonella* by means of a specific bacteriophage. J. Lab. Clin. Med. *44*, 51.

DACK, G.M. 1956. Food Poisoning, 3rd Edition. Univ. of Chicago Press, Chicago.

ENLOE, C.F., JR. 1967. A salmonella by any other name. Nutr. Today *2* (3) 11.

GALTON, M.M., SMITH, W.V., McELROTH, H.B. and HARDY, A.V. 1954. Salmonella in swine, cattle, and the environment of abattoirs, J. Infect. Dis. *95*, 236.

GALTON, M.M. *et al.* 1955. Salmonellosis in poultry and poultry processing plants in Florida. Am. J. Vet. Res. *16*, 132.

GANGAROSA, E.J. *et al.* 1968. Epidemic of febrile gastroenteritis due to *Salmonella java* traced to smoked whitefish. Am. J. Public Health *58*, 14.

HOROWITZ, M.A. and GANGAROSA, E.J. 1976. Foodborne disease outbreaks traced to poultry, United States 1966–1974. J. Milk Food Technol. *39*, 859.

KAUFFMAN, F. 1972. Serological Diagnosis of *Salmonella* Species, Kauffman-White-Schama. Williams & Wilkins Co., Baltimore.

LAMM, S.H. *et al.* 1972. Turtle-associated salmonellosis. I. An estimation of the magnitude of the problem in the United States 1970–1971. Am. J. Epidemiol. *95*, 511.

MacCREADY, R.A., REARDON, J.P. and SAPHRA, I. 1957. Salmonellosis in Massachusetts, sixteen-year experience. N. Engl. J. Med. *256*, 1121.

MacKENZIE, M.A. and GAINS, B.S. 1976. Dissemination of *Salmonella* serotypes from raw feed ingredients to chicken carcasses. Poultry Sci. *55*, 957.

McCLUNG, L.S. 1945. Human food poisoning due to growth of *Clostridium perfringens (C. welchii)* in freshly cooked chicken. J. Bacteriol. *50*, 229.

MORSE, E.V. and DUNCAN, M.A. 1974. Salmonellosis—an environmental health problem. J. Am. Vet. Med. Assoc. *165*, 1015.

NATL. ACAD. SCI. 1969. An evaluation of the *Salmonella* problem. Natl. Acad. Sci. Publ. *1683*.

NATL. COMMUNICABLE DIS. CENT. 1967. U.S. Public Health Serv., Atlanta, *Salmonella* Surveillance Rep. *67*.

PETHER, J.V.S. and GILBERT, R.J. 1971. The survival of Salmonellae on finger tips and transfer of organisms to food. J. Hyg. Cambridge *69*, 673.

ROSENSTEIN, B.J. 1967. Salmonellosis in infants and children: epidemiologic and therapeutic considerations. J. Pediatr. *70*, 1.

RUBENSTEIN, A.D., FEEMSTER, R.I. and SMITH, H.H. 1944. Salmonellosis as a public health problem in wartime. Am. J. Public Health *34*, 841.

SAPHRA, I. and WINTER, J.W. 1957. Clinical manifestations of salmonellosis in man. An evaluation of 7779 human infections identified at the New York Salmonella Center. N. Engl. J. Med. *230*, 1128.

SCHROEDER, S.A. 1967. What the sanitarian should know about salmonellae and staphylococci in milk and milk products. J. Milk Food Technol. *30*, 376.

SCHROEDER, S.A., ASERKOFF, B. and BRACHMAN, P.S. 1968. Epidemic salmonellosis in hospitals and institutions; a five-year review. N. Engl. J. Med. *279*, 674.

SCHROEDER, S.A., TERRY, P.M. and BENNETT, J.V. 1968. Antibiotic resistance and transfer factor in *Salmonella*, United States. J. Am. Med. Assoc. *205*, 903.

SMITH, E.R. and BRADLEY, B.W.D. 1971. Treatment of *Salmonella* enteritis and its effect on the carrier state. Can. Med. Assoc. J. *104*, 1004.

SWANSON, R.C. 1970. Household pets and salmonella. FDA Pap. (July-Aug.) 15.

3

Typhoid Fever

In the past when the occurrence of gastrointestinal diseases among children and adults was accepted as a way of life, it was said that one could tell the degree of sanitation of a community by looking at its typhoid rate.

Typhoid fever for centuries was confused with typhus fever and was known as "typhus abdominalis," until Louis, the distinguished French clinician in 1829, and William Gerhard of Philadelphia named it typhoid fever and distinguished it from typhus fever. William Budd in 1836 pointed out that typhoid fever is transmitted by the patient's excreta and stated that: "The living human body, therefore, is the soil in which this specific poison breeds and multiplies."

In the United States about 350,000 cases of typhoid fever, with 35,000 deaths, occurred in 1900, and in 1933 there were 65,000 cases also with a 10% case fatality rate. Today there still occurs an occasional case or a small limited outbreak in some areas.

The sanitary improvement of the environment and the prompt correction of any sanitary defect has resulted in the marked reduction and, in some areas, complete obliteration of one of the more severe intestinal infections. To elaborate, such favorable conditions have been brought about through the protection of the water supply, the sanitary disposal of sewage, the pasteurization of the milk supply, the supervision of the collection and marketing of shellfish from approved sources, the periodic sanitary inspection of food processing and serving establishments, and the education of their employees in personal hygiene and hand washing.

The few cases that still occur are caused by the ingestion of an item of food prepared or handled by a chronic typhoid carrier who is often located in the patient's own household. Occasionally, infection results while on a visit to places with substandard sanitation with illness occurring on returning home.

Characteristics

Typhoid fever is a systemic infectious disease characterized by continued fever, malaise, anorexia (loss of appetite), slow pulse, the involvement of lymphatic tissues with particular ulceration of Peyer's patches in the small intestine, enlargement of the spleen, cutaneous rose spots on the trunk, and diarrhea or constipation. Its infectious agent is *Salmonella typhi*, a mobile, flagellated, Gram-negative bacillus. V_i-phage tests have distinguished a number of types. Early in the disease, typhoid bacilli are found in the blood. They appear in the feces, and occasionally in the urine, after the first week. The agglutination reaction becomes positive during the second week.

Sources of Infection

As in the case with most of the other gastrointestinal diseases, man serves as the reservoir of infection, the disease being spread by patients and carriers. The incubation period of typhoid fever is from 1 to 3 weeks, but it usually is 2 weeks after the ingestion of the contaminated food or water. Patients discharge typhoid bacilli in their feces from the first week of illness throughout convalescence. About 10% may become transient carriers, shedding the bacilli for about 3 months after onset. Between 2 and 5% of patients will continue to discharge bacilli in their feces or urine for over 1 year and are thus declared to be chronic carriers. The rate is 3 to 5 times as high among infected females 40 to 49 years of age. These persons usually will harbor the organisms in their gastrointestinal tract for the rest of their lives. The bacilli frequently lodge in the gall bladder, infecting it and causing a cholecystitis. Often chronic carriers may go for periods of time with feces free of the bacilli, after which they start shedding them again.

Foods that favor the multiplication of typhoid bacilli and that are usually involved in the spread of typhoid fever are raw or inadequately cooked foods, or those that require no cooking such as raw vegetables and fruits, salads, pastries, unpasteurized milk and milk products, and shellfish from areas polluted by sewage. Contamination of food is usually by the fecal-soiled hands of a carrier or a missed case.

Flies are another source of spread by transferring typhoid bacilli from contaminated sewage to food. Water supplies, particularly from wells polluted by sewage from a neighboring cesspool containing the bacilli, have been incriminated in outbreaks.

Treatment

Typhoid fever may be treated with chloramphenicol taken orally every 6 hr until the temperature is normal, followed by smaller doses for 14 days. Ampicillin may be used, but it is not as effective.

Prevention

The occurrence of typhoid fever may be prevented in a community by application of the following measures: (1) the sanitary disposal of human excreta; (2) the protection, purification, and chlorination of the water supply; (3) adequate fly control by use of screening and spraying, as well as the elimination of fly breeding places such as accumulation of exposed garbage; (4) pasteurization or boiling of milk and milk products and supervision of commercial milk production; (5) periodic inspections and sanitary supervision of establishments where food is processed, prepared, and served; (6) prohibiting the collection and sale of shellfish except from approved sources; (7) instruction of patients convalescing from typhoid fever and chronic carriers in personal hygiene with emphasis on sanitary disposal of excreta and hand washing after defecation; (8) discovery and supervision of chronic typhoid carriers and their exclusion from working as food handlers; (9) health education of the general public and food handlers in the foodborne diseases, their sources of infection, and their modes of transmission; (10) vaccination of contacts and persons subject to unusual exposure.

Control of Infection Outbreak

Once a case or an outbreak of typhoid fever has occurred in a community, the following recommendations are made to control further spread:

(1) The health officer should be notified as promptly as possible.
(2) Hospitalization of patients is preferable to home care. In the latter case, the room should be fly-proof and a sanitary environment should be maintained.
(3) Feces and urine, as well as articles soiled therewith, should be disposed of or disinfected; bed linens and undergarments should be thoroughly laundered. With modern plumbing and adequate sewage disposal facilities, excreta may be disposed of directly into the flush toilet without preliminary disinfection.
(4) Milk should be pasteurized or boiled; water likewise should be chlorinated or boiled.

(5) A patient may be released from supervision by the health officer only when clinical symptoms have subsided and after 3 fecal and urine specimens submitted at least 24 hr apart are reported negative later than 1 month after onset. If any specimen in the series is positive, the patient may be released if negative cultures are obtained with 3 specimens at intervals of 1 month within the 12 months following onset.
(6) Family contacts should not be employed as food handlers until repeated cultures of feces and urine are negative indicating that they are not missed cases or carriers.

Epidemiologic investigation of all individual cases and outbreaks must be made as promptly as possible in order to determine the source of infection and introduce appropriate control measures. Each patient should be questioned regarding his whereabouts and places where he had consumed food outside of his home during a period of time coinciding with the incubation period of typhoid fever (2 to 3 weeks). Emphasis should be placed on such vulnerable foods as raw shellfish and raw milk and on water from suspicious sources. Histories are also obtained from all members of his household and from casual contacts as to any recent or past attack of gastroenteritis to determine whether there is a possibility of any of them being carriers. Fecal specimens are requested from all contacts for culture for typhoid bacilli in the laboratory. Should a contact be suspected from his history to be a chronic carrier, a blood specimen for V_i agglutination will prove helpful in confirming the suspicion. Phage typing of the typhoid bacilli isolated from the carrier's feces must be of the same type as that obtained from the patient in order to state with any degree of certainty that there is a causative relationship between the two.

Once the chronic carrier is identified, for the protection of the community he or she should be officially declared to be so and placed under restrictions similar to those specified in the New York State Sanitary Code [N.Y. State Health Counc. (undated)], which in part reads as follows:

(1) The urine and feces of a typhoid carrier shall be disposed of in such a manner that they will not endanger any public or private water supply or be accessible to flies.
(2) No typhoid carrier shall prepare or handle any food or drink to be consumed by persons other than members of the household with whom he resides.
(3) No typhoid carrier shall conduct or be employed in any restaurant, hotel, or boarding house, or conduct a lodging house in which, prior to taking lodgers, a separate toilet and bathroom have not been installed for the use solely of the

typhoid carrier, which toilet shall be located in a part of the house separate from any parts which may be occupied by a lodger.

(4) No typhoid carrier shall reside or be employed in a boarding home for children.

(5) No typhoid carrier shall engage in the occupation of nurse, cook, waiter, nurse-maid, or in any other occupation involving the handling of milk, cream, milk products, or utensils used in the production thereof.

If the carrier lives on a farm, then the following additional restrictions in the Sanitary Code apply to him:

No typhoid carrier shall be permitted to reside on premises on which one or more cows are kept except under conditions to be prescribed by the health officer, which conditions shall include a written agreement signed by the carrier, or if the carrier be a minor, by his parent or duly appointed guardian and by the owner of the cows or his representative. Such agreement shall stipulate either:

(a) that no milk, cream or other dairy products from such premises will be sold or given away to persons other than members of the household residing on such premises, or

(b) that milk and cream will be sold from such premises only after a special permit is issued by the local health officer and countersigned by the district state health officer and the local health officer of the jurisdiction in which the milk or cream is to be sold, provided, however, that a county health commissioner may issue such permit without the countersignature of the district state health officer. Such permit and agreement shall provide that:

(1) the milk or cream be sold only to the individual or firm designated in the permit, which individual or firm restricts its output to a pasteurized product.

(2) the carrier will not engage in any activities involving milking or handling of milk, cream or dairy utensils, or enter the milk house or barns where the milk-producing cows are kept.

(3) no milk or cream which is to be subsequently sold nor any utensils used in the production of milk or cream shall be brought into the house occupied by the carrier.

(4) no changes shall be made in the source of the water supply or in the system by which it is distributed on the farm, nor in the means of sewage disposal, except with the approval of the local health officer and the district state health officer.

(5) all other members of the carrier's household, except those who have had typhoid fever, shall have been vaccinated against typhoid fever.

The code also specifies that no typhoid carrier shall change his usual place of abode without first notifying the local health officer giving the proposed new address, and the health officer shall immediately inform the state department of health and the health officer into whose jurisdiction such a carrier is to remove.

One attack of typhoid fever confers a permanent immunity against a repeated attack. Immunization with a vaccine of high antigenicity should be administered to all household contacts in a primary series of 2 injections spaced several weeks apart, with a reinforcing injection given every 3 years. Recovered patients or carriers require no vaccination.

The epidemiologist visits the home of the carrier quarterly to ascertain that the instructions and restrictions are being carried out and to induce vaccination of any new member of the household. He is usually as welcome as the parole officer, since the carrier who is symptomless and appears to be in good health feels that he is being harassed and discriminated against by the health authorities.

To be declared a chronic typhoid carrier may result in great hardship. The carrier's occupation, if it is of the type enumerated in the Sanitary Code, must be changed without delay even though it results in unemployment. Familial and social problems have arisen in some instances once a person's carrier state has become known in spite of the confidential nature of such information. Adversity of this type has befallen several of the carriers discovered in the county after they have transmitted, usually unknowingly, the disease to contacts. One unhappy situation experienced by a newly-discovered carrier comes to mind. For a number of years a county resident had hoped and negotiated to bring her 60-year-old mother who lived in Turkey to the United States. When the mother was finally admitted, to the delight of the family, she took up residence in the household where she assisted with the housekeeping and cooking. About 4 months after her arrival, the daughter, her husband, and one of their children came down with typhoid fever. The mother was subsequently found to be a chronic typhoid carrier. As a result, filial love turned to enmity and the mother became a pariah. The daughter berated her and angrily ordered her out of the home and insisted she return to her native Turkey. The despondent mother, no doubt, would agree with King Lear (Act I, Scene 4), when he exclaimed, in despair, "How sharper than a serpent's tooth it is to have a thankless child!"

Epidemiologic Histories

A number of epidemiologic investigations of typhoid fever cases made by the author proved to be of extreme interest. A brief description of several of them follows.

Infection was reported in a young man living in a boarding house where he ate 2 meals a day prepared and served by his 60-year-old landlady who was found to be a chronic typhoid carrier. History revealed that she had had an attack of typhoid fever about 45 years previously and apparently had been a chronic typhoid carrier since. She had prepared meals for her boarders for 25 years, this allegedly being the first case she had ever caused. It seems that it had taken all that time for the circumstances necessary for the transmission of typhoid bacilli from her lower to the patient's upper digestive tract. In other words, on that critical day, if she was an intermittent carrier as is often the case, she had to be excreting the bacilli. She had to contaminate her hands following a bowel movement and fail to wash them. She then had to prepare food which was to be eaten uncooked (a tunafish salad in this case) and permit it to remain unrefrigerated long enough for the incubation of the bacilli. Apparently it had taken a quarter of a century for such a chain of circumstances to appear. If any one of the links in the chain had been missing at that time, the young boarder would have remained unattacked.

A young child came down with a severe case of typhoid fever. Fecal cultures from each household member, as well as from the parents of her playmate who occasionally offered the patient some goodies to eat, failed to disclose the carrier state in any of them. However, it was learned that about 2 weeks previous to the onset of illness, she had visited her grandmother who was bedridden and paralyzed following a stroke. The child had eaten some cookies while sitting on the grandmother's bed. Fecal specimens were obtained from the invalid, proving her on culture to be a chronic carrier. This illustrates the importance of including in the investigation all possible contacts, no matter how casual they may be.

Two girls, aged 8 and 14 years, residing in distant parts of the county developed typhoid fever about 24 hr apart. It was learned that they did not know one another and had had no known contact with each other. Both had recently returned from a visit to Canada, one traveling by train to Montreal accompanied by her grandmother, the other by automobile to Quebec with her father and sister. Members of each household were ruled out as carriers by history and fecal culture. A detailed itinerary of all the eating places visited was obtained from each parent. In comparing them for a common denominator, it was found that both children had been taken on the same day for a ride on the St. Lawrence River on the steamship *Tadousaac*. Further questioning revealed that the ship had 2 sources of water for the use of the passengers: a thermos carafe in each cabin containing drinking water and a wash basin over which a sign warned that the water (apparently pumped from the polluted river) was to be used only for washing. The younger child admitted drinking from the faucet, while the older girl stated that she only used the water to brush her teeth. The reporting of the findings to the state department of health resulted in the solution of the source of infection in a resident of Buffalo who had become ill following a Canadian visit. She also admitted having brushed her teeth aboard the *S.S. Tadousaac* on the same day as the two Nassau County cases. The Canadian Minister of Health was informed of these findings.

Two other small unrelated children residing several houses apart in one of the few slum areas in the county were reported to have typhoid fever with onsets several days apart. No carrier was found in either household. Sanitary inspection of the surroundings revealed an overflowing cesspool of a house located on an elevated area about a hundred yards away from the homes of the patients. The sewage had trickled down past a number of houses including those of the two children. In view of the critical unsanitary situation and the possible exposure of the community, it was felt advisable to set up a typhoid vaccination clinic in the school building on the premises at which nearly 100% of the residents of the area were immunized. Bacteriophage typing of the bacilli isolated from the feces of the 2 patients was reported by the New York State Department of Health Laboratory to be of a rare phage type only once before reported from typhoid bacilli isolated in Texas. With that information in mind, each resident was asked before being vaccinated whether he or she had ever visited or lived in Texas. One male stated that he had been employed as a chauffeur and that he and his employer had frequently visited Texas. He also said that he lived in the house on the hill with the overflowing cesspool. Although he could not recall any severe illness in the past, his V_i agglutination test was positive in an elevated titer and typhoid bacilli were isolated from his feces that proved to be of the same rare Texas type. Attention may be called to the epidemiologic significance in determining the phage type of isolated typhoid bacilli. If there is a history of contact and the bacilli isolated from the patient and the suspected carrier are the same phage type, a causative relationship may be assumed. On the other hand, should the phage types differ, then the epidemiologist must continue his search for a different carrier responsible for the infection. It may be said that phage typing is as important to the epidemiologist as fingerprints are to the criminologist.

On occasion, the epidemiologist may have to employ methods comparable to those used by the crime detective, as both are in search of a perpetrator—in the one instance an individual harboring a deadly weapon responsible for a crime, in the other a person harboring a virulent microorganism responsible for a disease. A case in point is a treasure hunt type of search made for a woman suspected of being a chronic carrier responsible for a primary and 3 secondary cases of typhoid fever in a household. She was a domestic who did housecleaning and laundry in the home of the patients and had access to the contents of the refrigerator so that she could prepare her own lunch. She could not be located as neither her surname nor her address was known to the patients. When it was learned that she did similar work in several homes in the neighborhood, a house-to-house visit was made until she was found ironing clothes in one of the homes. She was recognized as a known chronic typhoid carrier responsible for several cases of typhoid fever in her own and one other household. Like the notorious "Typhoid Mary," she had been placed under restrictions but had flagrantly disregarded them.

A 21-day-old baby girl was diagnosed as having typhoid fever. As the infant had been discharged from the hospital when she was only 5 days old, it was assumed that she had become infected in her home as no other case was traced to the hospital nursery. The mother was therefore suspected as being a chronic typhoid carrier and contaminating the baby's formula while preparing it. Cultures of the mother's feces confirmed that suspicion.

An outbreak of typhoid fever involving 72 children occurred in a summer day camp. After the water and milk had been eliminated as the vehicles responsible for the outbreak, culture of feces from the kitchen staff revealed the head cook to be a chronic typhoid carrier.

Fortunately today, with the occurrence of fewer cases of typhoid fever, carriers are not developing in sufficient number to offset the loss by death among the present older carriers. By the end of the century, if typhoid fever cases and outbreaks continue to be prevented and effectively controlled, all chronic carriers will have died, thus eliminating the last reservoir of infection in the country.

"Typhoid Mary"

The story of "Typhoid Mary" was the first of its kind to be reported in America, and it has become a classic. Mary was a cook in a family for 3 years and in 1901 she developed typhoid fever. At about the same time a visitor to the family had the disease. One month later, the laundress was taken ill.

Mary obtained a new position and 2 weeks after her arrival, the laundress became ill. A week later, a second case developed and soon 7 members of the household had come down with typhoid fever.

In 1904, she went to a home on Long Island that consisted of 4 persons and 7 servants. Within 3 weeks, 4 servants were attacked.

She then began cooking in 1906 for another family. Six members of the household of 11 developed typhoid fever between August 27 and September 3. By this time, the cook was first suspected. She entered another family on September 21 and on October 21, 1 of the domestics came down with typhoid fever.

In 1907, she again changed positions and entered a home in New York City. Two months after her arrival, 2 cases developed, 1 of which proved fatal. During these 5 years, Mary is known to have caused a total of 26 cases of typhoid fever.

She was virtually imprisoned by the New York City Department of Health in a hospital on March 19, 1907. Cultures taken every few days showed bacilli on and off for 3 years. Sometimes her feces contained enormous numbers of typhoid bacilli, and again for days none could be found.

Mary then escaped from observation until 1914 and in October of that year, she was engaged as a cook at the Sloane Hospital for Women in New York City. In January and February of 1915, an outbreak of typhoid fever occurred among 25 doctors, nurses, and other personnel of the institution. Mary was suspected but she left on a few hours leave and did not return or leave her address. She was, however, located by the health department under an assumed name.

A subsequent study of her career showed that she had infected still other persons beyond those already mentioned, and that she may have given rise to the well known waterborne outbreak of typhoid fever in Ithaca, N.Y., in 1903 involving over 1300 cases. The fact is that a woman bearing her name had been employed as a cook in the vicinity of the place where the first case appeared and from which contamination of the water supply occurred.

REFERENCES

BENENSON, A.S. 1970. Control of Communicable Diseases in Man. American Public Health Assoc., New York.

BRYAN, F.L. 1973. Diseases transmitted by foods. Cent. Dis. Control, Atlanta, Dep. Health, Educ. Welfare, CDC Publ. 73, 8237.

BUCHANAN, R.E. and GIBBONS, N.E. 1974. Bergey's Manual of Determinative Bacteriology, 8th Edition. Williams and Wilkins, Baltimore.

CRAUN, G.F. and McCABE, I.J. 1973. Review of the causes of waterborne disease outbreaks. J. Am. Water Works Assoc. 65, 74.

FARMER, J.J. and SIKES, J.V. 1974. Bacteriophage typing of Salmonella typhi in the United States: 1966–1973. Center for Disease Control, Atlanta, Salmonella Surveillance Rep. 119.

GREENBERG, M. 1943. The significance of the Widal reaction in enteric diseases in children. J. Pediatr. 23, 150.

MAXEY, K.F. and FOSENAU, M.J. 1965. Preventative Medicine and Public Health, 9th Edition. P.E. Sartwell (Editor). Appleton-Century-Crofts, New York.

N.Y. STATE HEALTH COUNC. (Undated). Control of Typhoid Carriers. Chapter 2. N.Y. State Sanitary Code, Albany, Reg. 33.

RUCKER, W.C. 1916. William Budd. Bull. Johns Hopkins Hosp. 27, 208.

TARTAKOW, I.J. 1977. Casebook of a medical detective: A review of interesting cases. Nassau County Med. Cent. *4* (2) 65–73.

TOPLEY, W.W.G. and WILSON, G.S. 1964. The Principles of Bacteriology and Immunology, 5th Edition. William Wood & Co., Baltimore.

4

Staphylococcal Food Poisoning

The terms "food infection" and "food poisoning" are not synonymous and must be differentiated. In food infection, a microorganism such as *Salmonella* enters the gastrointestinal tract in contaminated food, multiplies, and attacks the intestinal tissues, causing illness. In food poisoning, a chemical agent (arsenic, cadmium) or a poisonous organic plant or animal (mushrooms, clams) or a toxin (staphylococcal, botulinal), present in the food before it is eaten causes an intoxication when it is consumed. The most common form of food poisoning in the United States is that caused by enterotoxin-producing *Staphylococcus*. In that type of food poisoning, the staphylococci present in the food multiply at room temperature and produce the enterotoxin which causes the poisoning. As the toxin is preformed in the food, illness occurs within a short period of time after ingestion (1 to 6 hr, usually 2 to 4 hr). The toxin is thermostable, that is, not subject to alteration or destruction by heat; therefore, the application of heat to food contaminated with enterotoxin-producing staphylococci will not prevent the ensuing food poisoning.

A food poisoning outbreak may be differentiated from one caused by an infectious disease by its short incubation period and its explosive nature, the majority of cases occurring more or less simultaneously. The symptoms presented by the patients and the determination of the mean incubation period of the outbreak are most important as they give the epidemiologist a working hypothesis as to the causative agent. Should vomiting occur within minutes after ingestion, the most probable cause is a chemical poison; if illness appears 1 to 3 hr after the meal, a preformed bacterial enterotoxin may be suspected; if abdominal cramps, fever, vomiting, and diarrhea result within 1 to 3 days, *Salmonella* should be considered as the most probable etiologic agent. If neurologic rather than gastrointestinal symptoms, such as double vision and difficulties in swallowing, speech, and respiration, occur within a day or two, botulism must be given immediate consideration and specific antitoxins administered.

The other significant foodborne diseases, such as the dysenteries, typhoid fever, trichinosis, and infectious hepatitis, have more prolonged incubation periods. Of course, laboratory examination of the incriminated food, if available, and of fecal specimens obtained from patients is imperative in establishing a final diagnosis.

Characteristics

An individual case of staphylococcal food poisoning is often not recognized as its violent symptoms may be mistaken for those of an acute surgical abdomen requiring surgical exploration. However, it is easily recognized when illness occurs among a group of individuals who have come down with similar symptoms shortly after having partaken of the same food.

In order for a case or an outbreak of staphylococcal food poisoning to occur, the following conditions must be present:

(1) Inoculation: The contamination of a food with enterotoxin-producing staphylococci.
(2) Growth medium: A suitable food in which the organisms may multiply and produce the toxin.
(3) Incubation: Keeping the contaminated food for a suitable time period at a temperature compatible with the growth of the organism.

Illness is characterized by its sudden onset, with salivation, severe nausea and vomiting, retching, abdominal cramps, and diarrhea with occasional prostration. The incubation period and the severity of illness depend upon the amount of enterotoxin consumed and the susceptibility of the individual. Symptoms may appear within 1 hr, and in extreme cases, blood and mucus may be seen in the vomitus or feces. Often subnormal temperature and lowered blood pressure occur. In most instances recovery is prompt, the duration of illness being 1 or 2 days. Laboratory recovery of large numbers of enterotoxin-producing staphylococci on culture of suspected food and/or vomitus is usually diagnostic.

Sources of Infection

Among the foods most susceptible to staphylococcal contamination are pastries, custards, salads, chopped or sliced meats, ham, and bacon. Food may be contaminated with pus from a food handler's infected finger or abscess on an exposed part, or by nasal secretions. Staphylococci may even be present on hands with normal skin. Contaminated milk from a cow with mastitis (an infected udder), as well as milk products (cream, cheese) may also serve as sources of infection.

Prevention

Staphylococcal food poisoning may be prevented by the prompt refrigeration of all foods and leftovers, thus eliminating the incubation of any enterotoxin-producing staphylococci that may be present in the food. If the refrigerated food containing the staphylococci is eaten before the toxin has been formed, no illness will result.

The importance of the refrigeration of food cannot be overemphasized. Food prepared a number of hours before it is eaten should either be refrigerated at a temperature below 7.2°C (45°F) or kept heated above 65.5°C (150°F). Temperatures between these levels may be considered to be in a danger zone for the storage of food. The maximum length of time that cooked food may be kept between these temperatures should be 3 hr.

The occurrence of an outbreak of staphylococcal food poisoning among the guests at a wedding party held at a local hotel illustrates this point beyond any doubt. A sufficient quantity of chicken à la king (turkey was substituted) was prepared that morning in the hotel kitchen for 110 guests at a luncheon party and 185 guests at the wedding dinner to be served at 7 P.M. After lunch, the remaining creamed turkey preparation was permitted to remain at room temperature until the evening when it was placed in the steam heater and served to the wedding guests. None of the luncheon guests became ill. However, 131 or 78% of the wedding guests came down with severe gastroenteritis. Apparently, enterotoxin-producing staphylococci were introduced into the food during its preparation when the cooked turkeys were boned and cut up on the same cutting bench on which the raw birds had been eviscerated. The contaminated food was then kept at incubation temperature for a period of about 7 hr, during which time the microorganisms multiplied and produced their thermostable enterotoxin.

A number of staphylococcal food poisoning outbreaks have been found to be caused by contaminated custard-filled pastries exposed at room temperature in store showcases. It is recommended that bakers subject custards, just prior to their sale, to heat so as to destroy the staphylococci before they produce their toxin.

Persons with pyogenic skin lesions or with upper respiratory infection should be excluded from handling food. Kitchen employees assigned to the preparation of salads should wear disposable gloves. It is important to educate food handlers regarding this precaution, to point out the importance of cleanliness and sanitation of their kitchens, and the significance of proper refrigeration of foods.

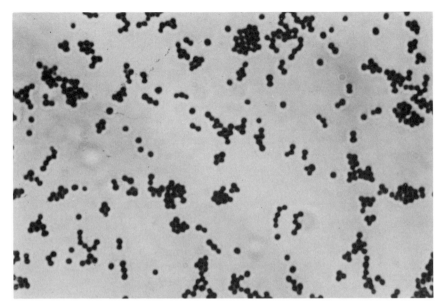

Courtesy of Elliot Scientific Corp. and Abbott Laboratories

FIG. 4.1. *STAPHYLOCOCCUS AUREUS.* GRAM STAIN OF SMEAR FROM CULTURE SHOWING TYPICAL "GRAPE-LIKE" CLUSTERS
May be in small groups, pairs, or short chains.

Diagnosis and Treatment

The assistance of the laboratory may prove helpful in determining whether an outbreak is caused by staphylococcal enterotoxin. The presence of extreme numbers of staphylococci in suspected food would indicate that the toxin, for which there is no chemical or bacteriological test available, is also present. Investigators have used such tests for the enterotoxin as feeding filtrates of cultures to human volunteers, or to monkeys, or injecting the filtrates into the abdomen or bloodstream of kittens or other animals.

If the contaminated food were heated after the enterotoxin was formed, the heat would destroy the bacteria but leave the toxin as capable of causing illness as before.

There is no specific treatment for staphylococcal food poisoning. As the vomiting tends to empty the stomach of its toxic contents and the diarrhea further eliminates the toxin from the intestinal tract, treatment for these conditions is unnecessary. If illness is severe, with shock, prostration, and low blood pressure due to loss of body fluids, normal saline solution parenterally is indicated.

Control

A survey of 95 outbreaks of staphylococcal food poisoning reported in the weekly communicable disease summaries issued by the U.S. Public Health Service in 1955 and 1956 was made by Hodge (1960). Completed data were also obtained from state, county, and city health officials who reported the incidents.

Analysis of the reports revealed that the determining factor in the development of staphylococcal food poisoning lies solely in keeping cooked protein food warm or at room temperature for 4 hr or longer. Of 83 fully reported outbreaks, the vehicles in 95% were cooked protein food which was subsequently kept unrefrigerated or warmed, or both.

Even though food may be handled cleanly by persons who are free of infection, the ubiquity of staphylococci among healthy persons ensures widespread contamination of food regardless of care of handling. Therefore recommendations for control of this disease have one objective: to prevent the staphylococci present in cooked protein food from producing enterotoxin.

INVESTIGATION OF OUTBREAK OF FOOD POISONING IN A DAY CAMP IN ROSLYN, N.Y.[1]

A report in detail of an investigation of a staphylococcal food poisoning outbreak is given. It is hoped that it will prove interesting as well as instructive. It may serve as a model to anyone who may have to make such an investigation.

An outbreak of food poisoning occurred on July 15 in a day camp located in Roslyn, New York. The camp is situated on approximately 3.2 ha (8 acres) upon which stand 2 frame buildings, 1 of which is a 4-story structure containing 22 rooms, and the other a combination garage and living quarters. Six rooms and the kitchen in the large building and the kitchen in the other building are utilized in the operation of the camp. It was established in 1945 and has functioned during the summer months, the present season having started June 30, and being expected to end August 23. The children reside in various parts of Nassau and Queens County and are transported to and from the camp in 4 large buses and 3

[1]Alexander D. Langmuir, M.D., Professor of Epidemiology, School of Hygiene and Public Health, Johns Hopkins University, has asked I. Jackson Tartakow, M.D., who made the investigation and prepared the report, for permission to use it for teaching purposes at the School of Hygiene and Public Health. In his letter, Dr. Langmuir stated: "I have been exceedingly interested in reading your very excellent and clear piece of work. I congratulate you on getting to the spot in the course of the epidemic itself. The only way to better your record would be to be present in advance of the outbreak, in which case you would be probably a patient also and not in shape to make an investigation."

station wagons. They arrive at 10 A.M. and leave for home at 4:30 P.M. Instructions are given in ballet dancing, art, dramatics, and swimming. The young group engages in supervised recreation.

At the time of the outbreak, the afternoon of July 15, Mrs. J.S., the director, reported by telephone that many of the children and personnel at the camp were retching and vomiting. She was greatly distressed and requested the help of the Department of Health. Investigation was started immediately.

Scope of Investigation

Attention was directed toward the following objectives:

(1) Obtainment of clinical histories from a large random sample of campers and personnel.
(2) Collection of data regarding the distribution of cases among campers by sex, age, and recreational groups or study classes.
(3) Determination of the articles of food and beverages consumed by the affected as well as unaffected individuals in the period of causation of the outbreak.
(4) Survey of conditions under which the foods were prepared, stored, and served.
(5) Submission of samples of food regarded as possibly implicated, as well as specimens of vomitus, stools, and nose and throat cultures for bacteriological examination; also chemical analysis of suspected food and vomitus.
(6) Study of factors which might have been instrumental in contamination of the foods, with special attention to means of preparation and storage of the foods served at the camp.

Clinical Character of Cases

Upon arrival at the camp, numerous children and several adults were seen lying on the lawn, some vomiting, others merely retching and salivating, most of them appearing distressed and a few in various degrees of prostration. Within the main building, children were on the floor and in beds, covered with blankets.

It was therefore possible for the investigator to observe for himself the objective symptoms and obtain direct information from those involved. Out of 101 individuals interviewed, 77 were ill. In general the clinical manifestations of these cases were similar. All complained of nausea and all but 1 vomited from 1 to 6 times. Abdominal cramps occurred in 58.4%, diarrhea (2 to 8 watery stools) in 35.1%, and prostration in 15.6%.

The frequency of other symptoms is shown in Table 4.1. Blood was noted in the vomitus of 1 patient.

The duration of the attacks ranged from 1 to 72 hr, but in most cases it was from 12 to 24 hr. In approximately 78% of the cases, illness was sufficiently disconcerting for the parents of the children involved to seek medical consultation. All recovered completely without any sequelae.

TABLE 4.1. FREQUENCY OF SYMPTOMS OF 77 CASES OF GASTROENTERITIS

| | Cases | |
Symptoms	Number	%
Nausea	77	100.0
Vomiting	76	98.7
Abdominal cramps	45	58.4
Diarrhea	27	35.1
Prostration	12	15.6
Chills	9	11.7
Fever	6	15.6

Incubation Period of Outbreak

Lunch was served between noon and 1 P.M. on July 15. The first case had its onset at 1:30 P.M. Over 75% of the cases became ill between 2:30 and 4:00 P.M., or from 2 to 4 hr after the meal. The onset of the last known case was at 10 P.M.

Number of Cases and Their Distribution

The outbreak was confined to the campers and the personnel. On the day of the outbreak, 181 children ranging in age from 4 to 14 years attended the camp. Of that number, 117 or 64.6% are known to have become ill. Illness was not limited to any class or recreational, sex, or age group. The personnel, which totaled 41, consisted of the owner and her assistant, 28 counselors and teachers, 4 bus drivers, a cook and helper, a maid, a caretaker, and several guests. Gastroenteritis occurred in 31 of the adults or 75.6%. The rate of recorded incidence for both the children and adults was 66.7% (Table 4.2). Difference in food habits or in susceptibility to the disease may account for the higher incidence rate among the adults.

TABLE 4.2. INCIDENCE RATE

| | Total Number | Attacked | | Not Attacked | |
		Number	Rate	Number	Rate
Campers	181	117	54.6	64	35.4
Personnel	41	31	75.6	10	24.4
Total	222	148	66.7	74	33.3

Possible Factors of Causation

The explosive character of the outbreak, the clinical manifestations, and the distribution of the cases suggested at the outset of the investigation that the outbreak was caused by food poisoning.

Water could be eliminated as a factor as its source is the Roslyn Water District which supplies an approximate population of 7000. Sewage is disposed via septic tank and tile fields, and does not endanger the water supply to the camp. No ice was used in drinking water or in any other beverage. Capped 1 qt (0.95 liter) bottles of milk in cases were kept cold by means of chunks of ice.

Contagion or personal contact between cases was precluded in view of the sudden onset and the distribution of the cases. Several of the personnel who had eaten no meals at the camp but were in close contact with those affected remained entirely exempt.

It therefore became apparent that food must have been the medium of conveyance of the causative agent, and the next step was to determine in what meal eaten within 24 hr of the onset of the outbreak the causative agent was spread. As the campers and counselors had been arriving daily at the camp at 10:00 A.M. and leaving at 4:30 P.M., the evening meal on July 14 and breakfast on July 15 were eaten at their respective homes. These 2 meals could therefore be dismissed from consideration as they had not been eaten in common at all, and no gastroenteritis had occurred among other members of the respective households.

It thus appeared that the luncheon, the only meal prepared at the camp and served to the campers and counselors on July 15, was definitely implicated. It was served in 3 shifts—at noon, 12:30, and 1:00 P.M.—outdoors from a large table in a shaded area adjoining the cottage or garage building, and was eaten in 3 dining rooms each seating from 20 to 30. A number of children and counselors ate their food outdoors on the lawn. The menu consisted of potato salad, sliced ham, bread and butter, butterscotch pudding, and milk.

The milk was obtained from the Borden Company that morning and delivered in well-capped 1 qt (0.95 liter) bottles in cases. Chunks of ice, supplied by the milk company, were placed on top of the bottles in order to keep the milk cold. The cases were kept outdoors in the shade. Milk was served from the quart bottles in individual service paper cups.

The ham was "Polish Style" canned boiled ham. Three cans, each weighing about 10 lb (0.45 kg), were purchased on the morning of July 15 from H.C. Bohack Company store in Roslyn Heights, N.Y. The cans were opened at the store by one of the butchers and the hams were sliced on the mechanical slicer. The man who handled the hams appeared in good health, had no skin eruptions on the hands, arms, or face, and stated that he had had no recent sore throat or gastroenteritis. The sliced meat was taken to the camp where it was placed, in its wrapping, on the outdoor service table. It remained unrefrigerated from 10:30 A.M. until it was served between 12:00 A.M. and 1:00 P.M.

The bread and butter sandwiches consisted of slices of Wonder Bread, "Pullman Loaf," buttered just before lunch with half butter and half Nucoa. The butter and margarine mixture had been kept refrigerated previous to its use.

The butterscotch pudding was prepared at 3:00 P.M. on July 14 in the kitchen of the large house. It was made with a prepared mix known as "Butterscotch Flavor Dessert, Regal Gold Banner Brand," manufactured by Regal Food, Inc., New York, N.Y. Sufficient quantities of the mix, canned "Pet" evaporated milk, water, and brown sugar were used to make about 20 qt (18.9 liters) of pudding. When it started to boil, the pot with the pudding was removed from the stove and the contents poured into a 5 gal. (18.9 liter) iron can. After cooling at room temperature, the can was covered and stored on the floor of the laundry room in the basement. It remained there unrefrigerated until 10:00 A.M. the following day when it was taken to the outdoor table. It was served in paper cups at lunchtime. At no time was the dessert refrigerated. The temperature of the laundry room at the time of the investigation was about 21°C (70°F).

The potato salad was also prepared on July 14, the day previous to the outbreak. Beginning at 1:00 P.M., 100 lb (45.4 kg) of unpeeled potatoes were boiled in water. While still hot, the skins were removed by the cook and helper. The potatoes were then placed in a large can made of galvanized sheet iron—the type commonly used for the storage of garbage or ashes. The can was then covered with a cover of the same metal, and at about 4:00 P.M. was taken down to the laundry room by 2 counselors and placed next to the smaller can of pudding. On July 15 at 9:30 A.M. it was taken to the outdoor kitchen. The potatoes were then sliced by the cook and helper, and mixed with cut-up hard boiled eggs (2 dozen boiled that morning), celery, onion, and parsley (from Bohack). A mayonnaise dressing as well as additional oil (Mazola), vinegar (Bohack), and salt were then worked thoroughly with a large metal spoon into the potato mixture in the galvanized can.

The dressing was taken from an unopened jar which was labelled "Heller's Red Seal, Pure Mayonnaise," manufactured by Venice Importing Company, Brooklyn, N.Y. It contained oil, eggs, vinegar, sugar, and spice; the oil, upon inquiry from the manufacturer, was found to be soybean oil. The preparation of the salad was completed at about 11:00 A.M. It remained outdoors and was served on paper dishes and eaten 1 to 2 hr later. The potato salad, like the butterscotch pudding, was not refrigerated.

Among a random sample of 101 individuals interviewed, everyone who was attacked in the outbreak gave a history of having eaten some of the potato salad; no one who had not eaten the salad became ill (Table 4.3). Of that group, 81 stated that they had eaten potato salad, and 77 of them became ill, giving an attack rate of 97.0%. Of the 24 who were not attacked, only 4 ate some salad.

TABLE 4.3. PERCENTAGE OF ATTACKED AND UNATTACKED INDIVIDUALS WHO ATE DIFFERENT FOODS SERVED AT LUNCH ON JULY 15

Foods Served	Percentage of Individuals Eating Different Foods	
	Attacked %	Not Attacked %
Potato salad	100.0	16.7
Ham	96.1	75.0
Bread and butter	93.5	75.0
Pudding	58.4	50.0
Milk	85.4	83.3

The pudding, in spite of the unsatisfactory temperature under which it was stored, could be eliminated as a factor as only 58.4% of those attacked ate it and 50% of those who remained well partook of it.

The epidemiologic evidence alone definitely established (a) the outbreak as due to food poisoning, (b) the noonday luncheon as the meal in which the causative agent of the outbreak was distributed, and (c) the potato salad as the sole medium of conveyance.

Mode of Contamination

The question as to how the potato salad became contaminated then arose. It may have been by human hands, by flies, roaches, mice or other vermin, by utensils, or through the air.

The sanitary and hygienic conditions in the kitchens of the main house and cottage in general appeared satisfactory. Refrigeration facilities, however, were inadequate, an 11 ft^3 (0.33 m^3) refrigerator being used to store food eaten by approximately 225 persons. A soil line running through a room in the basement was found to contain a 5 cm (2 in.) opening from which a fixture had apparently been removed. The wall and floor showed evidence of sewage having overflowed through this opening. The storage and disposal of garbage was found to be unsatisfactory as no covered cans were used and incompletely burned paper plates and food were found on the ground.

Flies, roaches, mice, or rats were not in evidence. A professional exterminator makes periodic visits to the camp and buildings and keeps insects and rodents under control.

The salad was prepared and served by the cook and her assistant. Previous to the outbreak, both were in good health and free from any infections of the respiratory or gastrointestinal tracts. The cook had several small healing wounds of the hands, the result of cuts inflicted in the course of her work. Although these injuries did not appear infected, they may have harbored pathogenic microorganisms. The boiled potatoes which she peeled on July 14 may or may not have become contaminated in this manner. The cook stated that on the morning of July 15, while cutting up the boiled potatoes, she ate one and found it to be "still warm"—excellent incubation conditions.

Inspection of the large galvanized sheet iron can which was used to store the boiled potatoes and the prepared potato salad revealed it to be totally unsuitable as a container for food. It was constructed in such a manner that numerous creases, seams, and crevices could have lodged particles of food. Washing, no matter how thorough, could not dislodge all the food in the crevices. Examination of the empty and "cleaned" can confirmed this conclusion. An odor of spoiled food was evident from the can which allegedly had been washed with hot water and soap powder.

Infective Agent

According to Dack (1956), the time intervals present between the eating of incriminated food and the beginning of gastrointestinal symptoms due to various specific agents has been found to be as follows: botulism, average 1 to 2 days; staphylococcus enterotoxin, 1 to 6 hr, average 2½ to 3 hr; *Salmonella*, 7 to 72 hr, average 12 to 24 hr; *Streptococcus* (alpha type), 5 to 18 hr.

The short incubation period, the relative mildness of the symptoms, and the rapid recovery tend to rule out botulism as well as *Salmonella* and *Streptococcus* as the causative agent.

The short interval between the eating of the potato salad and the onset of symptoms is evidence that the outbreak was caused either by a poison or a preformed toxin, rather than a bacterial infection which requires time for multiplication in the intestinal tract before infection is manifest.

Solanine poisoning could be eliminated by epidemiologic history. This type of poisoning, several outbreaks of which are found in the literature, is caused by an alkaloid which is normally present in potato in insignificant amount, but may occur in toxic doses in green sprouting or shrivelled potatoes. No illness was reported by other persons in the county who ate potatoes from the same source.

Poisoning due to chemical coating with which the galvanized can might have been treated at the factory was ruled out. The can was purchased on July 2, and potato salad was prepared and stored in it on the following day. It had been used on 2 other occasions without anyone who had partaken of the foods becoming ill. The last time the can had been used was on July 11 for the preparation and storage of lettuce and cabbage salad.

The acidity of the salad due to the vinegar made it necessary to rule out as a factor zinc or antimony poisoning from the galvanized coating of the can. Callender and Gentzkow (1937) reported acute poisoning of 2 companies of soldiers from drinking limeade prepared in galvanized iron garbage cans similar to the one used in this instance.

Chemical poisoning due to accidental introduction of an insecticide or rodenticide into the salad had to be given consideration even though no such chemicals could be found on the premises. This was ruled out by laboratory examination.

The findings in this outbreak appear to conform with the conditions outlined by Dack (1956) as necessary for an outbreak of *Staphylococcus* food poisoning:

(1) Contamination of a food with an enterotoxin-producing strain of *Staphylococcus*: In this instance the peeled boiled potatoes were most likely contaminated by hands, spray from the nose or throat, or by organisms present in the unsanitary galvanized can.
(2) A suitable food in which *Staphylococcus* can grow and produce enterotoxin: Starch media are excellent for the growth of *Staphylococcus*; according to *Bergey's Manual* (Buchanan and Gibbons, 1974), *Staphylococcus* grows abundantly on potato.
(3) Keeping the food for a sufficient period of time at a temperature compatible with growth: The boiled peeled potatoes were kept at room temperature for about 18 hr.

Laboratory Findings

It is rather unusual for an investigator to be summoned to the scene of a food poisoning outbreak while it is still in its second act. Ordinarily he learns of it after the curtain has come down and pertinent evidence has been either discarded or destroyed and important information forgotten. The arrival of this investigator at the locale of the outbreak within an hour of its onset made it possible for him to obtain specimens of potato salad, mayonnaise dressing, vomitus, feces, and nose and throat cultures for bacteriological and chemical examination.

Food.—The findings in the New York City branch of the State Department of Health in the bacteriological examination of samples of food included: (1) presence of *Staphylococcus aureus* as the predominating organism in the potatoes (*Bacillus subtilis* and *Escherichia coli* were also isolated); (2) absence of *Salmonella* organisms from the potatoes and the salad; (3) absence of any significant microorganisms from the mayonnaise dressing. The cultural examination was made from the inner portion of several chunks of potato in the salad rather than from their surface, thus implicating the potatoes and eliminating the mayonnaise dressing, celery, eggs, and the other ingredients of the salad as the medium of conveyance of the causative agent.

Chemical analysis of the potato salad at the laboratory of the New York Station of the Food and Drug Administration showed no heavy metals, arsenic, or fluoride present. The mayonnaise dressing, examined by the Technical Research Laboratory of the Nassau County Police Department, failed to show the presence of arsenic.

Vomitus.—Three specimens of vomitus obtained from 2 campers and 1 counselor on July 15 were reported as containing no microorganisms of diagnostic significance by the state branch laboratory, and no heavy metals, arsenic, or fluoride by the laboratory of the Food and Drug Administration.

Feces.—Specimens of feces submitted by the cook and 2 campers, all of whom had diarrhea at the time of the investigation, were examined in the state branch laboratory and found negative for typhoid, dysentery, and paratyphoid bacilli or other species of *Salmonella.*

Nose and Throat Cultures.—*Staphylococcus aureus* of the same strain as that found in the potatoes was isolated from cultures taken from the throat and nasopharynx of the cook and assistant cook.

Of especial significance was the finding in the potatoes of *Staphylococcus aureus* in large numbers and the absence of other kinds of organisms found in food poisoning. *Escherichia coli* and *Proteus vulgaris* in this instance were believed to be secondary invaders and did not play any significant role in the food poisoning. The failure to find staphylococci in the vomitus of individuals who had ingested the salad containing the microorganism and its enterotoxin suggests that although the preformed toxin remains sufficiently potent to cause gastrointestinal irritation, the microorganism itself is destroyed by the gastric acidity.

The isolation of *Staphylococcus aureus* from the upper respiratory tract of the individuals who handled the potatoes and prepared the salad may be a highly significant factor, making contamination by means of droplets from the nose and throat appear probable. In a study of the sources of foodborne outbreaks in war industry, Getting *et al.* (1944) report the following:

"Our study demonstrates that staphylococcal food poisoning outbreaks may be traced to specific food handlers as sources of infection. In each instance where it was possible to culture the nose and throat of persons responsible for the preparation of an incriminated product, an apparently identical strain of *Staphylococcus aureus* was recovered from at least one of the food handlers and the infected food. Although staphylococci are a universal contaminant of the environment, those strains harbored in the nose and throat of the food handlers are invariably associated with outbreaks."

Laboratory facilities (feeding to kittens and intravenous kitten injection test) for determining whether the staphylococci isolated were of an enterotoxigenic strain were not available to this investigator. An attempt, however, was made to determine whether the staphylococci isolated from the food handlers and from the potatoes were identical.

Potatoes and potato salad have previously been incriminated in outbreaks of gastroenteritis. Dieudonne reported illness in 150 to 180 persons allegedly caused by potato salad infected with *Proteus vulgaris* (Tanner 1933). An outbreak caused by mashed potatoes infected with *Escherichia coli communior* in which 100 persons were affected was reported by Jansen and den Dooren de Jong (Tanner 1933).

Summary

An outbreak of food poisoning occurred in a day camp among the campers (ages 4 to 14) and personnel on July 15. Out of 181 campers and 41 personnel, 66.7% became ill.

The clinical manifestations of the cases were in general very similar with nausea, vomiting, and abdominal cramps predominant. Diarrhea occurred in only 35.1% of those attacked.

The epidemiologic evidence obtained incriminated potato salad, specifically the potatoes, which were boiled and peeled on the previous day and kept unrefrigerated for about 18 hr, as the medium of conveyance of the agent which caused the outbreak.

The short interval between the eating of the salad and the beginning of the outbreak, the relative mildness of the symptoms, and the rapid recovery tend to indicate that the causative agent was in all probability a preformed enterotoxin such as that produced by *Staphylococcus aureus*.

The finding of this microorganism in large number in potatoes of the salad tends to support the epidemiologic evidence.

The food handlers who prepared the salad were found to be carriers of *Staphylococcus aureus*.

Conclusion

(1) The medium of conveyance of the agent causing the outbreak was potato salad served at the noon meal on July 15.

(2) The causative agent was apparently a bacterial toxin produced by an enterotoxigenic strain of *Staphylococcus aureus.*

(3) The potatoes became contaminated with staphylococci after they were boiled, most probably while they were being peeled. The microorganism may have been present in the crevices and seams of the unsanitary galvanized sheet iron can in which they were stored, or may have been introduced by human hands, or floating droplets from the nose and throat of 1 of the 2 food handlers, both of whom were found to be carriers of that organism.

(4) Tremendous multiplication of the infecting organisms in the potatoes with formation of the enterotoxin occurred during the 18 hr period the cooked potatoes were kept unrefrigerated. This long incubation period was probably responsible for the high attack rate of 97.0%.

(5) The following recommendations were made to the manager of the camp as a safeguard against the recurrence of such an outbreak:

   (a) Installation of adequate refrigeration facilities so that food prepared for the campers and personnel may be properly stored at a temperature below 7.2°C (45°F).

   (b) Slicing or similar handling of all food should be done as soon as possible before actual serving.

   (c) Use of proper cooking utensils for the preparation and covering of containers for the storage of food.

   (d) Food handlers with infections of the skin, nose, or throat, or a recent history of diarrhea should not be permitted to participate in the preparation or serving of food.

   (e) Instructions should be given to food handlers on the importance of personal hygiene, with special emphasis on keeping the hands away from the mouth and nose, covering the mouth with a handkerchief while coughing or sneezing, and proper handwashing after visiting the toilet.

   (f) Correction of existing unsanitary conditions (garbage storage and disposal, repair of broken soil line in basement, proper handwashing facilities in toilets).

REFERENCES

BENENSON, A.S. 1975. Communicable Diseases in Man, 12th Edition. American Public Health Association, Washington, D.C.

BERGDOLL, M.S., REISER, R. and SPITZ, J. 1976. Staphylococcal enterotoxin detection in food. Food Technol. *30* (5) 80.

BRYAN, F.L. 1976. Public health aspects of cream-filled pastries. A review. J. Milk Food Technol. *39*, 289.

BUCHANAN, R.E. and GIBBONS, N.E. 1974. Bergey's Manual of Determinative Bacteriology, 8th Edition. Williams & Wilkins Co., Baltimore.

CALLENDER, G.R. and GENTZKOW, C.J. 1937. Acute poisoning by the zinc and antimony content of lemonade prepared in a galvanized iron can. Mil. Surg. *80*, 87.

DACK, G.E. 1956. Food Poisoning, 3rd Edition. Univ. of Chicago Press, Chicago.

GETTING, V.A., RUBENSTEIN, A.D. and FOLEY, G.E. 1944. Staphylococcus and streptococcus carriers; sources of foodborne outbreaks in war industry. Am. J. Public Health *34*, 883.

GILBERT, R.J. 1974. Staphylococcal food poisoning and botulism. Postgrad. Med. J. *50*, 607.

HODGE, B.E. 1960. Control of staphylococcal food poisoning. Public Health Rep., Public Health Serv., U.S. Dep. Health, Educ. Welfare *75* (4) 355.

PAYNE, D.N. and WOOD, J.M. 1974. The incidence of enterotoxin production in strains of *Staphylococcus aureus* isolated from foods. J. Appl. Bacteriol. *37*, 319.

SCHROEDER, S.A. 1967. What the sanitarian should know about salmonellae and staphylococci in milk and milk products. J. Milk Food Technol. *30*, 376.

TANNER, F.W. 1933. Foodborne Infections and Intoxications. Twin City Printing Co., Champaign, Ill.

TATINI, S.R. 1973. Influence of food environments on growth of *Staphylococcus aureus* and production of various enterotoxins. J. Milk Food Technol. *26*, 559.

TROLLER, J.A. 1976. Staphylococcal growth and enterotoxin production—factors for control. J. Milk Food Technol. *37*, 449.

Botulism

In a small town in South Dakota on September 14, 1936, a country hotel keeper, his wife, and 3 boarders sat down to a meal consisting of potatoes, boiled bologna sausages, home-canned string beans, bread, butter, and coffee. On opening the mason jar in which the string beans had been canned by the cold-pack method, the landlady noted that they were slightly foamy and faintly rancid in odor. When she questioned their edibility, one of the boarders assured her that they would be all right if rinsed off in cold water. She did this and served them. When the platter of beans was passed to 1 of the other boarders, he detected a rancid odor, "somewhat like limburger cheese but not strong enough to be offensive," so he did not take any. He was the only one of the group who ate none of the beans but ate heartily of all the other foods. He was also the only 1 of the 5 to remain alive and well 42 hours later.

This is abstracted from a report by Hunter *et al.* (1940). As an editorial note, it may be added that had the string beans been brought to a boil before serving them, instead of rinsed with cold water, although their taste might have been unsavory, death from botulism poisoning of the other 4 diners would have been prevented.

Characteristics

The microorganism that causes botulism, *Clostridium botulinum*, is a harmless saprophyte, but the toxin it produces is one of the most potent poisons known to mankind. Botulism differs from other types of food-borne diseases in that it attacks chiefly the central nervous system with only minor gastrointestinal symptoms.

Like the enterotoxin-producing *Staphylococcus*, it is the toxin and not the bacillus that causes the illness. It differs from the staphylococci in that the fatality rate of staphylococcal food poisoning is, for all practical purposes, negligible, while that of botulism is about 65% and higher when large quantities of the neurotoxin are ingested and absorbed.

Botulism was known in Germany during the 19th century as "sausage poisoning." Hence it got its name from *botulus*, Latin for sausage. It was subsequently found that it was also caused by other underprocessed foods, such as smoked meat and fish, and canned vegetables and meats.

Botulism is a serious intoxication. It is caused by a rod-shaped spore-forming anaerobic bacillus that produces a neurotoxin that is absorbed and attacks the cranial and other motor nerves. The illness it causes is sometimes preceded by acute digestive disturbances (nausea, vomiting, and constipation) within 12 to 24 hr after ingestion of contaminated food. This may be accompanied by weakness, dizziness, headache, and muscular uncoordination. It is soon followed by signs of paralysis of the cranial nerves with diplopia (double vision), blepharoptosia (narrowing of the slit between the eyelids), mydriasis (dilation of pupils) and loss of pupillary light reflex, hoarseness with difficulty in speech and in swallowing, with paralysis of pharyngeal muscles and regurgitation through the mouth and nose in fatal cases. Temperature and blood pressure may remain normal throughout the illness. Due to the inability to swallow, signs of aspiration pneumonia may occur and prove fatal. Death is usually due to respiratory or cardiac failure. It is fortunate that today botulism is a relatively rare disease.

There are 7 different types of *C. botulinum*, but only types A, B, E, and F cause disease in man. The degree of the specificity of each type is such that antitoxin for 1 type will not neutralize the toxin of another type. Types A and B are most common in the United States, although occasionally, as in fish poisoning, type E is encountered (Fig. 5.1). Attacks are usually either in individual cases or in family groups that partake of a food so prepared or preserved as to permit toxin formation.

Sources of Infection

The toxin is formed by the vegetative cells of *C. botulinum* under anaerobic conditions, usually in nonacid protein foods. Unlike the toxin produced by staphylococci, botulinus toxin is thermolabile (destroyed by heat). Higher temperatures, however, are required for the inactivation of the spores. Spores are widely distributed. Their reservoir of infection is soil, and they are also found in dust, water, and in the animal intestinal tract.

Illness may occur within 12 to 16 hr after eating food containing the toxin. The incubation period may be considerably shorter with a more severe illness, with death occurring within 3 to 6 days if the ingested food contains a high concentration of toxin. On the other hand, it may take several days for symptoms to appear should the dose of toxin be minimal, as it may be with acid foods or those with little nutrient value for the growth of *C. botulinum*. The spores cannot germinate at a pH less than 4.8.

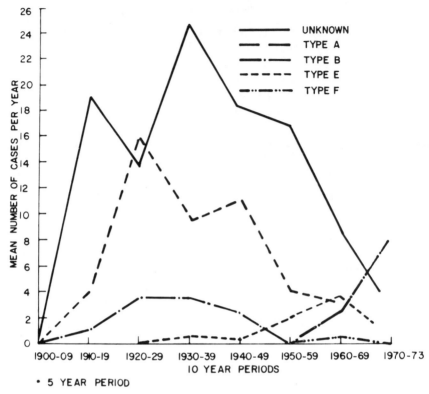

From Cent. Dis. Control (1977)

FIG. 5.1. THE NUMBER OF CASES OF BOTULISM IN THE UNITED STATES BY TYPES OF TOXIN, 1900–1973

The disease occurs in persons who have ingested contaminated food from cans, jars, or sealed plastic containers inadequately processed during canning and eaten without preliminary heating. With few exceptions, cases and outbreaks of botulinus food poisoning have been seen during wartime when food is being conserved and people are doing a great amount of home canning. Cases have been traced to improper canning of vegetables, meats, and meat products, fish and seafood, and other protein foods, preserved, pickled, or otherwise processed. The heat often used in home cold-pack canning may not be sufficient to kill the spores and inactivate the toxin. That is the reason that the pressure cooker method is recommended, as a temperature of 120°C held for 10 min is necessary to destroy both toxin and spores. Low acid foods (pH greater than 5.0) and medium acid foods (pH 4.5–5.0) should be processed at temperatures of 120°C or greater.

Usually food invaded with *C. botulinum* and its toxin may have an abnormal odor, appear gassy or foamy, and have a sharp or acid or bitter taste, thus warning individuals that the food is spoiled and it would be the height of folly to eat any of it. Unfortunately, in some instances, in spite of its lethal potentiality, there may be no change in odor or taste, thus giving the consumer no hint of its danger.

Dack (1956) reports a survey made by K.B. Meyer in which there were 462 botulinus outbreaks in the United States and Canada between 1899 and 1947. With very few exceptions, the outbreaks were caused by foods that were home canned.

Commercially canned products are rarely responsible for botulinus poisoning as such foods are subjected to proper sterilizing heat previous to marketing. It is conceivable, however, that temperature controls in a processing plant may become temporarily impaired permitting incompletely processed foods to reach the market.

Occasionally a single can of commercially canned food may be incriminated through no fault of the processor. Although the can had left the factory in satisfactory condition, it may have subsequently become dented or may have fallen to the floor, resulting in a small opening in its seam sufficient to permit botulinus spores present in soil and dust to enter the can. With the escaping food drying and sealing off the opening in the can, the spores that have entered will grow in the can's anaerobic atmosphere and produce the deadly toxin. In 1971 a New York man and his wife came down with botulism after eating the contents of a can of Bon Vivant Vichyssoise soup. The man died and although the woman had signs of paralysis and had to be tracheotomized, she survived by the administration of antitoxin.

Diagnosis and Treatment

If food containing botulinus toxin is fed to chickens, they develop limber-neck and die. In the laboratory, testing for the toxin and determining its type is made by grinding the suspected food plus sterile sand in a mortar with saline solution, centrifuging it, and injecting the supernatant liquid intraperitoneally into a series of mice, each of which has been previously protected with a different type of antitoxin (A, B, and E). The surviving mouse is the one that had received protection against the toxin in question. In other words, if the mice immunized against toxins B and E die but the one that received antitoxin A survives, then it may be assumed that type A toxin is responsible for the case or outbreak, and the patient(s) should be promptly given type A antitoxin.

The sooner the determination of the type involved is made and the proper antitoxin administered, the more favorable the prognosis of the persons involved. Delay in diagnosis, laboratory examination, and treatment may prove fatal because of the absorption of the toxin and its irreparable damage to the tissues. If prompt laboratory testing is not available, polyvalent botulinus antitoxin (A, B, and E) may be used. Contacts who ate the incriminated food must also be immunized within 36 hr. Antitoxins are available from the National Communicable Disease Center in Atlanta, Georgia.

Control

Individual cases and outbreaks of botulism must be reported to the health authorities so that action may be taken in determining the cause of infection, finding the food responsible for the illness, and arranging for the immunization of contacts. If a commercially canned product is involved, a recall action is instituted by the responsible regulatory agency. Sanitarians are instructed to visit the food markets to embargo cans with the same code number as the one on the incriminated can(s), and to deliver one or more unopened cans to the laboratory for examination. The manufacturer and distributors of the food in question are contacted by local, state, or federal agencies in order to learn how widely the food has been distributed. Occasionally the manufacturer becomes aware of the situation and voluntarily institutes a recall action before notifying the health agency.

As has been stated, botulism is very rarely caused by commercially canned or processed foods as such plants are under governmental control through regulations and inspections. As most cases result from improper home canning, it is important to educate homemakers in safe methods such as timing, pressure, and temperature required to destroy botulinus spores and of the necessity of boiling all home-canned vegetables for 10 min before serving.

One wonders whether Moses Maimonides, Court Physician to Saladin, Sultan of Egypt during the 14th century, when foods were preserved by drying and salting, was aware of botulism when he wrote:

There are some foods which are extremely detrimental and it is proper for man never to eat them, such as large salted old fish, old salted cheese, truffles, mushrooms, old salted meat, wine must, and a cooked dish which has been kept until it acquired a foul odor. Likewise any food whose odor is bad or excessively bitter is like a fatal poison unto the body.

REFERENCES

ARNON, S.S. et al. 1977. Infant botulism. Epidemiological, clinical and laboratory aspects. J. Am. Med. Assoc. 237, 1946.

BENENSON, A.S. 1975. Control of Communicable Diseases in Man, 11th Edition. American Public Health Association, Washington, D.C.

CENT. DIS. CONTROL. 1977. Foodborne and Waterborne Disease Outbreaks. Annual Summary 1976. Center for Disease Control, Atlanta.

COMMUNICABLE DIS. CENT. 1974. Botulism in the United States 1899–1973. Handbook for Epidemiologists, Clinicians and Laboratory Workers. U.S. Dep. Health, Educ. Welfare, Center for Disease Control, Atlanta.

DACK, G.M. 1956. Food Poisoning, 3rd Edition. Univ. of Chicago Press, Chicago.

DOLMAN, C.E. and AGER, E.A. 1964. Type E botulism. J. Am. Med. Assoc. *187*, 538.

GILBERT, R.J. 1974. Staphylococcal food poisoning and botulism. Postgrad. Med. J. *50*, 603.

HAYNES, S., CRAIG, J.M. and PILCHER, K.S. 1970. The detection of *Clostridium botulinum* type E in smoked fish products in the Pacific Northwest. Can. J. Microbiol. *16*, 207.

HUHTANEN, C.N., NAGHSKI, J., CUSTER, C.S. and RUSSELL, R.W. 1976. Growth and toxin production by *Clostridium botulinum* in moldy tomato juice. Appl. Environ. Microbiol. *32*, 711.

HUNTER, C.A., WEISS, J.E. and OLSON, C.L. 1940. Outbreak of botulism. Lancet *60*, 67.

KOENIG, M.G. *et al.* 1964. Clinical and laboratory observations of E botulism in man. Medicine (Baltimore) *43*, 517.

KOENIG, M.G. *et al.* 1967. Type B botulism in man. Am. J. Med. *62*, 208.

MAXEY, K.E. and ROSENAU, M.J. 1965. Preventive Medicine and Public Health, 9th Edition. P.E. Sartwell (Editor). Appleton-Century-Crofts, New York.

SMITH, L.D.S. 1977. Botulism. The Organism, Its Toxins, the Disease. Charles C. Thomas, Springfield, Ill.

U.S. DEP. HEALTH, EDUC. WELFARE, PUBLIC HEALTH SERV. 1973. Botulism in the United States, 1899–1973. Center for Disease Control, Atlanta.

6

Shigellosis

Characteristics

Shigellosis or bacillary dysentery is an acute infection of the bowel with frequent diarrhea often streaked with blood, mucus or pus, fever, vomiting, abdominal cramps, and tenesmus (ineffective efforts at defecation). In severe cases there is marked dehydration and abdominal distention It is most severe in infants (25% fatality) and children (5% fatality). It occurs most frequently in the tropics and is seen where there are overcrowding, poor sanitary conditions, and malnutrition. Outbreaks have occurred in institutions for children, in jails, in mental hospitals, in military camps, and on Indian reservations.

Its infective agent is the *Shigella* bacillus named after Shiga, the Japanese observer who found it responsible for dysentery in his country. The bacillus has many serotypes and is divided into 4 groups: (1) *S. dysenteriae*, (2) *S. flexneri*, (3) *S. boydii*, (4) *S. sonnei*.

Dysentery cases and outbreaks in the United States are usually caused by *S. sonnei* and *S. flexneri*. The incubation period is 1 to 7 days, usually less than 4 days. The disease is self-limiting and complications (except in infants and children) are rare.

Sources of Infection

Like most of the other intestinal diseases, it is spread by fecal-oral transmission by man or by domestic animals harboring the bacilli in their feces, and by contaminated food or water. It may also be spread by inanimate objects soiled with feces. Flies acting as mechanical vectors can transmit the bacilli from infected fecal material to food. Dysentery is transmitted by patients during the acute phase of the disease until their feces no longer contain the organism. This usually takes several weeks but occasionally the carrier state occurs with recovered patients shedding *Shigella* bacilli in their feces for a year or two.

Prevention

With improved sanitation, dysentery has become an infrequent disease in developed countries. Its prevention may be maintained, as in the case of typhoid fever, through sanitary disposal of human feces, by the protection and purification of the water supply, by the pasteurization of milk and dairy products, and by the sanitary supervision of the processing, preparation, and serving of foods. As infants and children are most vulnerable to the disease, it is important to educate mothers in the hygiene of breast feeding and the preparation of formulas, with emphasis on the boiling of milk and water. As in the other foodborne diseases, handwashing after defecation and before handling of food must be carried out. It is also important to protect foods against contamination by flies through screening and fly control.

Control

As in typhoid fever, the occurrence of cases or outbreaks must be reported to the health authorities, particularly if the outbreak occurs in a school or institution, so that an investigation may be made and control measures recommended. Patients should be placed under rigid precautions to prevent fecal spread. A search should be made among the contacts for mild or unrecognized cases. Contacts should not be permitted to work as food handlers until 3 negative fecal cultures at daily intervals are reported. The patient must be kept under surveillance until his feces are shown to be free of *Shigella* bacilli.

Treatment

The patient may be treated with antimicrobial drugs (tetracycline, chloramphenicol, or ampicillin). Some strains of *Shigella* have become resistant to the sulfonamides. The dehydration and loss of electrolytes (sodium, potassium, etc.) must be corrected with large amounts of water, milk, and other fluids, especially in the treatment of infants and young children. The patient's garments should be soaked in soap and water followed by boiling. Spread by flies should be prevented by the screening of the home and the use of mosquito netting.

An excellent illustration of the spread of shigellosis by flies is given in the report of the following investigation made by the author.

INVESTIGATION OF OUTBREAK OF SEVERE GASTROENTERITIS IN MEN OF 101ST INFANTRY, U.S. ARMY, WHILE ON BIVOUAC

Reason for Investigation

It was learned indirectly that there were 8 cases of severe gastroenteritis admitted to the hospital at the U.S. Army Post at Mitchell Field, located in Nassau County, N.Y. Although it was known that the army took care of its own sick personnel and was not under any obligation to report cases or outbreaks to the civil health authorities, the assistance of the department of health was offered in the investigation of the outbreak, the determination of its cause, and the recommendation of control measures. The offer was readily accepted by the medical officer in charge.

Investigation

A visit was made to the post hospital and it was learned from the medical inspector at the post that the illness had been diagnosed as bacillary dysentery on the basis of fecal examinations. All were members of the 101st Infantry Company with headquarters at Bethpage, N.Y. They were out on bivouac for field experience. The patients were interviewed and the information obtained is given in Table 6.1.

It may be seen that 2 patients (F.G. and P.K.) give a history of having had a similar illness a year before, and another patient (C.B.) had a severe attack of gastroenteritis about 6 months previously. It is conceivable that any of these 3 men may have had a previous attack of dysentery and may have been a chronic carrier responsible for the presence of *Shigella* in the contents of the latrines. Relapse and reinfection are known to occur.

The peak of this rather limited outbreak may be said to be August 22 and 24 with 2 cases occurring on each of these days. Diarrhea, cramps, and fever appear to be the most consistent symptoms in all the cases. Fecal specimens had been examined at the post hospital laboratory and *S. flexneri* was isolated from all 8 specimens.

In going over the environmental conditions at the bivouac grounds, it was learned that the camp consisted of about 800 enlisted men divided into 5 companies. Each company had its own kitchen with 8 men detailed to it.

Kitchens.—Four of the kitchens were of the outdoor type consisting of merely a wood platform and a canvas top. Only 1 kitchen was completely

TABLE 6.1. CASES OF DYSENTERY ACCORDING TO AGE, DATES OF ONSET, HOSPITALIZATION, AND SYMPTOMS

| Name | Age | Date of Onset | Date of Hospitalization | Signs and Symptoms | | | | | | | | |
				Diarrhea	Nausea	Vomiting	Fever	Cramps	Chills	Headache	Previous Attack
L.P.	21	8-14-42	8-17-42	6–10×	0	+	+	+	0	0	0
F.G.	27	8-18-42	8-28-42	+	+	0	+	+	+	+	8-41
C.B.	32	8-22-42	8-31-42	2–3×	+	0	+	+	+	0	2-42
S.L.	25	8-22-42	8-27-42	6–20×	0	+	+	+	0	0	0
P.K.	21	8-23-42	8-25-42	4–8×	+	0	+	+	0	0	8-41
G.K.	21	8-24-42	8-24-42	20×	0	0	+	+	+	+	0
J.C.	27	8-24-42	8-25-42	+	0	0	+	+	0	0	0
J.L.	22	8-28-42	8-28-42	Bloody	+	+	+	+	0	+	0

screened. Food was served and eaten outdoors. The fly infestation in and around each kitchen was very great. At lunchtime during the distribution of food, flies were seen to alight continually upon it. Although many flies were present outside the screened kitchen, very few were seen inside. Fly traps were placed outside the kitchens but they were inadequate as they caught very few flies. All 8 patients ate their food from unscreened kitchens.

Latrines.—Numerous latrines scattered over the camp grounds were inspected and found to be in unsatisfactory condition. They were open and a number of the seats were not covered due to broken hinges. The latrines were heavily infested with flies. At some points, the soil at the sides had caved into the pits leaving openings at the base for flies to enter and leave.

Food Handlers.—None of the men working in the kitchens had had chronic dysentery. An attempt to search out a chronic carrier among them through fecal examination proved unproductive.

Milk Supply.—The milk served was Borden's pasteurized, purchased in 1 qt (0.95 liter) bottles and kept refrigerated in regulation ground ice-boxes.

Water Supply.—The water used at the camp was from the Central Park Water District which is approved and serves that area.

Conclusions

In view of the abundance of files present both in the kitchens and the latrines, it is reasonable to conclude that the food prepared and eaten at the camp was contaminated by the flies. It may be assumed that a carrier of shigellosis was present at the camp and that his excreta, mixed with that of other members, is the source of infection. The flies contaminated the food when they commuted from the latrines to the open kitchens, depositing the *Shigella* bacilli that were on their legs and bodies that they had picked up during their first visit. The fact that none of the men who had eaten food from the screened kitchen had become ill tends to substantiate this conclusion.

Recommendations

The following control measures were recommended to the medical inspector:

(1) Screening of all kitchens.
(2) Fly-proofing the latrines and closing openings at their bases.
(3) Repairing the covers of the latrine seats.
(4) Using adequate fly traps and fly paper in the kitchens.
(5) Attempting to find carriers and undiagnosed cases through repeated bacteriological examination of feces of men with persistent diarrhea.

REFERENCES

BENENSON, A.S. 1970. Control of Communicable Diseases in Man, 11th Edition. American Public Health Association, Washington, D.C.

COMMUNICABLE DIS. CENT. 1977. *Shigella* Surveillance Rep. *39*. Annual Summary 1976. Center for Disease Control, Atlanta.

KIMBALL, A.M., THACKER, S.B. and LEVY, M.E. 1980. *Shigella* surveillance in a large metropolitan area. Assessment of a passive reporting system. Am. J. Public Health *70*, 164.

LEVINE, M.M. *et al.* 1973. Pathogenesis of *Shigella dysenteriae* I. (Shiga) dysentery. J. Infect. Dis. *127*, 261.

MAXEY, K.E. and ROSENOW, M.J. 1965. Preventive Medicine and Public Health, 9th Edition. P.E. Sartwell (Editor). Appleton-Century-Crofts, New York.

TARTAKOW, I.J. 1977. Casebook of a medical detective: A review of interesting cases. Nassau County Med. Cent. *4* (2) 65-73.

TOPLEY, W.W.C. and WILSON, G.S. 1964. The Principles of Bacteriology and Immunology, 5th Edition. William Wood & Co., Baltimore.

7

Streptococcal Food Infection

Two types of streptococci are known to cause illness when their portal of entry to the human body is the gastrointestinal tract. The types are: (1) Alpha-type *Streptococcus faecalis* (Lancefield Group D) and (2) *Streptococcus pyogenes* (Group A, hemolytic). Food infection results when the ingested food is contaminated with *S. faecalis*. On the other hand, food that contains *S. pyogenes* has a greater affinity for the respiratory than for the digestive tract. It is capable of causing a variety of diseases, among them streptococcal sore throat, scarlet fever, erysipelas, and puerperal fever, as well as localized infections such as cellulitis, lymphadenitis, mastoiditis, otitis media, peritonitis, septicemia contagiosa, and various skin and wound infections.

Characteristics

Gastroenteritis caused by *S. faecalis* is more or less a mild infection dependent upon the concentration of microorganisms in the ingested food. The incubation period is from 2 to 18 hr, and the symptoms consist of nausea, vomiting, diarrhea, and abdominal cramps. Illness is much milder than in staphylococcal food poisoning and is of shorter duration.

Alpha-type *S. faecalis*, which is a natural inhabitant of the intestinal tract of man and various animals, must be ingested in enormous quantities to cause illness, as many people have different degrees of immunity to such infection. However, outbreaks involving numbers of persons have been reported and confirmed by laboratory examinations. The foods incriminated have been beef croquettes, sausage (canned Viennese), ham, bologna, turkey dressing, coconut cream pie, and whipped cream.

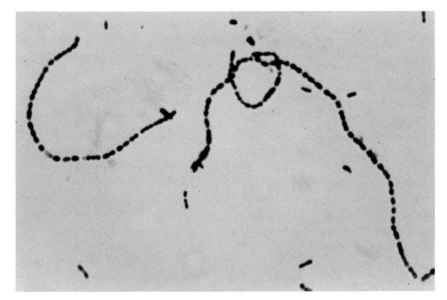

Courtesy of Elliot Scientific Corp. and Abbott Laboratories

FIG. 7.1. STREPTOCOCCI. GRAM STAIN OF CULTURE WITH LONG CHAIN FORMA-
TION

Sources of Infection

The diseases that are caused by *S. pyogenes* (Group A) are transmitted
to the respiratory system by intimate contact with patients or carriers,
through the inhalation of droplets containing the organisms, or by the
ingestion of milk or other foods contaminated with that organism. The
foodborne disease usually caused by *S. pyogenes*, often occurring explo-
sively in outbreaks, is streptococcal sore throat. It is considered to be a
form of scarlet fever without the skin rash (exanthem), as the streptococci may fail to produce the erythrogenic toxin, or the infected person
because of a previous attack may be immune to the toxin.

Symptoms and Diagnosis

Patients usually complain of nausea and vomiting, fever, sore throat, an
exudative tonsillitis or pharyngitis with injection and edema, tender
cervical lymph nodes (adenopathy), headache, and muscular pains. Final
diagnosis is made by the isolation of *S. pyogenes* from a throat culture. In
severe cases, complications such as otitis media, peritonsillar abscess,

acute glomerulonephritis, or rheumatic fever may occur. Fatality from streptococcal sore throat is low, with only 1 death per 300 to 400 cases.

The disease has an incubation period of 1 to 3 days. The acutely ill or convalescent patient and the carrier serve as its reservoir of infection. In the uncomplicated case, infection may be transmitted for about 10 days, but the carrier state may in some instances last for months.

Treatment

As *S. pyogenes* (Group A) is known to come in at least 40 serologically distinct types, each with its specific immunologic characteristics, it is possible for individuals to suffer repeated attacks of streptococcal sore throat, with each infection being caused by a different type. Treatment is with chemotherapy (penicillin, or erythromycin if sensitive to penicillin). It should be started promptly in order to prevent the occurrence of complications.

Laboratory facilities should be provided in available areas so that physicians and public health officers may submit specimens for the isolation of streptococci and for serologic typing.

Prevention

The incidence of streptococcal sore throat may be appreciably reduced by educating the public in its modes of transmission and its relation to its complications. As in the prevention of the other foodborne diseases, if milk is not pasteurized, then it should be boiled; milk from cows with mastitis should not be used or sold; food handlers as well as other persons having an upper respiratory infection or other septic condition should be excluded from the preparation or serving of food. Foods which favor the growth of streptococci (such as deviled eggs) should be prepared just before serving or should be refrigerated at 5°C at (41°F) or below.

Control

Cases or outbreaks should be reported to the health officer for reasons already stated. Infected persons should be isolated for 7 days or longer from the time of onset in order to protect contacts. However, if the patient is receiving treatment with penicillin, isolation may be terminated after 24 hr and treatment should be continued for 10 days. Contacts or persons who have partaken of the incriminated food should be given penicillin prophylactically.

In the event of an outbreak it is of extreme importance to promptly determine the source of infection and manner of spread. Special attention should be given to the possibility of raw milk's being involved.

Before the pasteurization of milk was universally practiced, an out-break of scarlet fever involving 840 persons occurred in Boston in 1910. The patients were customers on the dairy route of a large milk contrac-tor. The source of the infection was traced to a "missed case" of scarlet fever on one of the farms that supplied raw milk to the contractor. Pasteurization promptly checked the outbreak.

A report of the investigation of a foodborne outbreak of streptococcal sore throat that occurred in Nassau County follows.

REPORT OF INVESTIGATION OF SEPTIC SORE THROAT OUTBREAK

Reason for Investigation

On the morning of May 20, Dr. I.F. reported the occurrence of sore throat, septic in character, in 5 women. He further stated that these patients had all attended a church luncheon on May 17th, and he believed that there were more cases to be found.

Investigation—An investigation was made on May 20 and 21 to determine the source of infection:

1. *Attendance.*—It was learned that a group of 117 women residing in Rockville Centre, Freeport, Baldwin, Merrick, Bellmore, and Hempstead, N.Y., attended a benefit luncheon held at Temple Israel, Freeport, on May 17.

The 5 women treated by Dr. I.F. were interviewed, and a list of food items eaten by them was obtained. Cultures of their throats were taken and sent to the New York State Branch Laboratory for examination.

2. *Preparation of Food.*—The food for the luncheon was purchased, prepared, and served by a committee of women consisting of 11 mem-bers, the caretaker of the Temple, and his wife. The chairman of the luncheon committee, Mrs. S.G., was visited; she submitted a list of the members of the committee who participated in the handling of the food. She also checked the membership list of the women who attended the luncheon.

3. *Menu.*—The menu included the following items: canned tomato juice, poured directly from the can into paper cups; egg salad made by chopping hard boiled eggs and mayonnaise with minced green peppers and celery. Mayonnaise was taken directly from a freshly opened glass jar. The egg salad was served on leaves of lettuce with sliced tomatoes and shredded fresh carrots. A ball of cottage cheese mixed with chopped walnuts and sour cream was placed on each plate. Small rolls and butter, coffee and

evaporated milk from freshly opened cans mixed with homogenized pasteurized milk from containers, and honey buns baked by 2 committee members completed the menu. With the exception of the cake, the food was purchased from local grocery stores by various committee members.

Samples of the egg salad and cheese and nut salad were not available for laboratory examination. Samples of the mayonnaise, however, used in the preparation of the former were obtained and cultured at Meadowbrook Hospital, and reported negative for hemolytic streptococci on June 8.

4. *Food Handlers.*—All the members of the committee, the caretaker and his wife (total 13 individuals), and a sample of 40 guests were interviewed. Throat cultures were taken from 9 committee members regardless of whether or not each had been ill. The caretaker, C.S., and his wife, Mrs. S.S., who had assisted in the kitchen with the dishes and had set the tables and washed the cooking utensils, were also cultured. Mrs. S.S. gave a history of sore throat, fever, and "grippe-like" feeling beginning the morning of May 17, the day of the luncheon. She denied handling any of the food either during preparation or in serving it.

No definite duties had been assigned to any of the committee members, but all participated in the kitchen activities as the need arose.

Of the 13 food handlers, 9 became ill with sore throat, fever, malaise, and muscular pains (Table 7.1). The onset of illness was on May 18 and 19, 2 and 3 days, respectively, after the luncheon. Throat cultures of all 9 were positive for hemolytic *Streptococcus*, 3 of them being reported as belonging to "serologic Group A." Four persons were not ill and no hemolytic streptococci were isolated from their throats. The chairlady, Mrs. S.G., who was not ill, gave a history of having had an infected ingrown toenail incised the morning of the luncheon and having changed the dressing several times that day. On examination on May 20 and 21 the incision appeared completely healed and no drainage was observed. However, culture from her throat was reported positive for hemolytic streptococci, Group A. She claimed that she had not handled the food to any extent, with the exception of boiling 13 dozen eggs and chopping the nuts on the evening previous to the luncheon. Although she denied shelling the eggs, 2 members of the committee claimed that several dozen were brought to the Temple already shelled—probably by Mrs. S.G. She also stated that she took home some egg salad which was eaten that evening by her husband and son. The latter became ill on May 18 with signs and symptoms of septic sore throat. The culture from her son's throat was reported positive for hemolytic streptococci, Group A. The husband complained of a "scratchy" throat and some malaise the same day.

TABLE 7.1. LUNCHEON COMMITTEE, FOOD EATEN, DATE OF ONSET OF ILLNESS, AND RESULT OF THROAT CULTURES

Name	Onset	Food Eaten							Culture for Hemolytic *Streptococcus*	Remarks
		Tomato Juice	Egg Salad	Cheese and Nuts	Vegetable	Coffee and Milk	Cake	Rolls and Butter		
S.G.	none	+	+	+	+	+	+	+	positive	not ill
B.T.	5/18	+	+	+	+	+	+	+	none	ill
I.W.	5/18	−	+	+	+	+	+	+	positive	ill
C.S.	5/18	+	+	+	+	+	+	−	none	ill
A.B.	5/19	+	+	+	+	+	+	+	positive	ill
B.K.	none	+	+	+	+	+	+	+	negative	not ill
M.G.	5/18	+	+	+	+	+	+	+	none	ill
R.S.	5/18	+	+	+	+	+	+	+	positive	ill
G.S.	none	+	+	+	+	+	+	+	negative	not ill
J.L.	none	+	+	+	+	+	+	+	negative	not ill
S.S.	5/17	+	+	+	+	+	+	+	positive	ill day of lunch
C.S.[1]	5/19	+	+	+	+	+	+	+	negative	ill
D.S.	not at home	—	—	—	—	—	—	—	—	—

[1] Only male in group; caretaker of Temple.

5. *Guests.*—A sample of 40 additional persons who were guests at the luncheon were interviewed; 21 of them became ill. All had eaten egg salad and all but 1 had the cheese and nuts. Three throat cultures were reported positive for hemolytic streptococci. Nineteen of the guests did not become ill; 18 of them ate both the egg and cheese salad.

Taken as a whole, 52 persons were interviewed; 33 (63.4%) became ill on May 17, 18, and 19; 19 (36.6%) women remained well. The greatest number of cases, 23, had their onset on May 18 (Table 7.2).

TABLE 7.2.   CASES ACCORDING TO DATE OF ONSET

| Date of Onset | Cases | |
	Number	%
May 17	1	3.0
May 18	23	69.7
May 19	9	27.3

6. *Clinical Symptoms.*—The most prevalent symptom was a painful throat, which occurred in all cases (Table 7.3).

Throat cultures from 13 individuals, 9 of whom became ill, were examined at the New York State Branch Laboratory, *Streptococcus pyogenes* being isolated from all. From the cultures taken on the 4 non-cases, 1 was reported positive (*Streptococcus pyogenes* Group A). This culture came from Mrs. S.C., chairlady of the committee.

TABLE 7.3. NUMBER OF CASES WITH SIGNS AND SYMPTOMS ACCORDING TO DATES OF ONSET

| Signs and Symptoms | Date of Onset | | | |
	May 17	May 18	May 19	Total
Painful throat	2	21	10	33
Fever	1	15	5	21
Headache	1	9	6	16
Muscular pains	1	7	5	13
Cervical adenitis	1	9	2	12
Exudate of throat	0	8	2	10
Nausea	0	1	1	2
Vomiting	0	1	0	1

7. *Attack Rates of Food Served.*—Epidemiologic analysis was made of the items on the menu eaten by the 52 persons interviewed. The egg salad was eaten by 100% of those who became ill, and by 94.7% of the non-cases. The cheese and nut salad was eaten by 90.9% of cases, and by 94.7% of the non-cases (Table 7.4).

TABLE 7.4. ATTACK RATES OF ITEMS ON MENU

| | Cases | | Non-cases | |
	Number	Attack Rate per 100	Number	Attack Rate per 100
Egg salad	33[1]	100.0	18	94.7
Cheese and nut salad	30	90.9	18	94.7
Cake	30	90.9	19	100.0
Vegetables	28	87.8	18	94.7
Tomato juice	28	84.8	16	84.2
Rolls and butter	28	84.8	18	94.7
Coffee and cream	28	84.8	19	94.7

[1] 3 persons ate egg salad taken home by members of the luncheon committee.

Summary of Findings

(1) Each of the cases of septic sore throat ate food at or intended for the church luncheon on the afternoon of May 17.

(2) The food was prepared that morning in the kitchen of the Temple and kept without refrigeration until it was eaten between 1:00 and 2:00 P.M.

(3) The milk supply was excluded as no cases of septic sore throat other than those who attended the luncheon were reported in the county on or about that time. The same may be said of the water supply.

(4) Each of the patients ate egg salad.

(5) The attack rate with the egg salad was 100% for those who became ill, and 94.7% for those who did not become ill.

(6) The attack rate with the cottage cheese and nuts was 90.9% for those who became ill, and 94.7% for those who did not become ill.

(7) The husband and son of one woman and the daughter of another became ill after eating a portion of the egg salad which had been taken home.

(8) The eggs were boiled and several dozen presumably shelled on the evening before the luncheon by Mrs. S.G., chairlady of the luncheon committee.

(9) The nuts used in the cottage cheese salad were chopped by Mrs. S.G. the evening before.

(10) The caretaker's wife, Mrs. S.S., assisted in the kitchen.

(11) Mrs. S.G. gave a history of having had an infected ingrown toenail incised by a podiatrist on the morning of the luncheon and having changed the dressing several times that day.

(12) Although she was not ill before or after the luncheon, culture of her throat was positive for hemolytic streptococcus Group A.

(13) Mrs. S.S. gave a history of sore throat and "grippy" feeling while assisting in the kitchen at the time of the luncheon.

(14) *Streptococcus pyogenes* Group A was also isolated from her throat.

Conclusion

Evidence seems to point to the egg salad as the most probable cause of the outbreak. It is probable that the causative organism *(Streptococcus pyogenes* Group A) was introduced into the salad by either:

(1) Mrs. S.G., chairlady of the luncheon committee
   (a) as a carrier (positive throat culture but no symptom), or
   (b) from the infected incised ingrown toenail (culture not obtained) or
(2) Mrs. S.S., caretaker's wife, as a case of septic sore throat (positive throat culture).

REFERENCES

BENENSON, A.S. 1975. Control of Communicable Diseases in Man, 12th Edition. American Public Health Association, Washington, D.C.

ESSELEN, W.B. and LEVINE, A.A. 1957. Bacterial food poisoning and its control. A review. Univ. Mass. Coll. Agric., Amherst, Bull. *493.*

LEAVEN, L.J. 1968. Foodborne epidemic of Group G streptococcal pharyngitis. Vt. Morbidity Mortality *17,* 406.

McCORMACK, J.S., KAY, D., HAYES, M. and FELDMAN, R.A. 1976. Epidemic streptococcal sore throat following a community picnic. J. Am. Med. Assoc. *236,* 1039.

SASLOW, M.S. *et al.* 1974. Outbreak of foodborne Streptococcal disease—Florida. Morbidity Mortality *23,* 365.

WILSON, G.S. and MILES, A.A. 1975. Streptococcal infections. *In* Topley and Wilson's Principles of Bacteriology and Immunology, Vol. 1 and 2, 6th Edition. Williams & Wilkins Co., Baltimore.

8

Cholera

Immigrants from Russia on their way to the United States in 1892, pending their embarkation, were temporarily housed in overcrowded barracks on one of the wharves along the Elbe River in Hamburg. Many of them came from districts in Russia where cholera outbreaks were occurring. Among the immigrants there unquestionably must have been some mild cases of cholera or at least some convalescent carriers. As the sewage of the permanent residents of Hamburg emptied into the Elbe River, that of the immigrants was likewise discharged at the wharf directly into the river. The city of Hamburg (640,000 population) and its adjacent town of Altona (142,000 population) both rest on the Elbe River and at that time their residents were furnished with drinking water from the polluted river. Altona, however, filtered its water by the slow sand process, while Hamburg's supply went untreated. As the result of the contamination of the river water, an epidemic of cholera occurred. This was confirmed by the isolation of the specific microorganism causing the disease, from both the feces of patients as well as the river water. It is interesting to note that although the residents of both communities drank the infected river water, the death rate in Hamburg was nearly 6 times that of Altona (134.4 per 10,000 population compared to 23.0 per 10,000). The small number of cases in Altona occurred along the boundary where the people had access to Hamburg's raw unfiltered water.

The description of the Hamburg cholera epidemic is given because it remains, together with "The Case of the Broad Street Pump" in London (see page 3), a classic in the archives of public health and environmental sanitation. The London outbreak demonstrated that an enteric disease like cholera may be transmitted by drinking water, and the Hamburg epidemic proved that a water supply contaminated with a pathogenic organism may be made potable if it receives adequate treatment. In this case it pointed out the effectiveness of filtering out cholera bacilli, thus giving impetus to slow sand filtration.

Four pandemics of cholera swept Europe between 1830 and 1875. The disease entered the United States in 1832 by way of New York and Quebec and reached west as far as the military post on the upper Mississippi. It was again brought to this country by transatlantic liner a year later through New Orleans and was spread west as far as California by the forty-niners in their search for gold. It prevailed widely in this country with cases appearing in New York City.

The most severe epidemic, which lasted more than 10 years and claimed millions of lives, occurred in India during the first quarter of the 20th century. Epidemics also appeared in Egypt and in the Philippine Islands. Thus the disease acquired the name of "Asiatic Cholera." Although it is considered to be a disease of the tropics, the ravages of cholera have been visited on most of the countries of the world as it spread along the routes of travel and trade.

Characteristics

Cholera is an acute specific infection characterized by a sudden onset of violent purging, vomiting, cramps, subnormal temperature, extreme dehydration, and circulatory collapse. It is caused by the *Vibrio cholerae* discovered by Robert Koch in 1883 and named the "comma bacillus" because of its shape. Cholera has a brief incubation period, from several hours to 3 days, rarely over 5 days. Fatality rate ranges between 30 and 80% with death sometimes occurring within a few hours after onset. Diagnosis may be confirmed by the presence of large numbers of comma-shaped bacilli on direct microscopic examination of a fecal or vomitus smear, and by isolation of the *Vibrio* on culture.

Source of Infection

As in typhoid fever, salmonellosis, and shigellosis, man is the reservoir of infection of cholera. When infected, he sheds the *Vibrio* in large numbers in his feces. The disease is spread when the feces or vomitus of patients or convalescent carriers contaminates food, milk, or water, the latter being its chief means of spread. Fruits and vegetables washed with contaminated water may convey the disease when eaten. It may also be spread by direct contact with patients or indirectly by flies. Most spread occurs early in the disease and occasionally during convalescence.

Prevention

During an epidemic, preventive measures are similar to those recommended for typhoid fever: sanitary disposal of patients' feces and vomitus, protection and purification of the water supply, pasteurization or boiling of milk and other foods, fly control, and education of the public in personal hygiene and hand washing. Prophylactic vaccination protects against the disease for about 1 year when specific antibodies begin to diminish in the bloodstream. Persons living in endemic areas often acquire immunity to cholera through minute inapparent infections.

Control

Cases of cholera must be reported to the health authorities. As the disease is extremely rare in the United States, when it arises it is imported from another country. Epidemics may have to be traced to their source in a foreign country by the World Health Organization. In order to prevent such importation by travelers, whenever a person comes from a country where cholera is endemic or epidemic, the United States Public Health Service notifies the health officer in his destination to keep him under surveillance for a period of 5 days (the longest incubation period of cholera) in order to ascertain that he is not incubating the disease on his arrival.

Treatment

Patients should be isolated during the acute stage of cholera. Scrupulous cleanliness, hand washing, and careful handling and disposal of vomitus, feces, and soiled linens must be observed by persons caring for the sick. Prompt parenteral therapy must be given, using adequate volumes of isotonic balanced electrolyte solutions to correct dehydration, acidosis, and hypokalemia, if the patient is in shock, very ill, or vomiting repeatedly. Otherwise, the solution is given by mouth. Tetracycline or other antimicrobial agents may shorten the acute phase of the disease. Family contacts should be treated prophylactically with vaccine or tetracycline.

The correction of imperfect sewerage and the prevention of the contamination of potable water supplies have made cholera a rarity in this country.

REFERENCES

BARUA, D. and BARROWS, W. 1974. Cholera. W.B. Saunders Co., Philadelphia.

BENENSON, A.S. 1975. Control of Communicable Diseases in Man. American Public Health Association, Wshington, D.C.

BLAKE, P.A. *et al.* 1977. Cholera in Portugal 1974. I. Modes of transmission. II. Transmission by bottled mineral water. Am. J. Epidemiol. *105*, 337.

BUSHNELL, O.A. and BROOKHYSER, C.S. 1965. Proceedings of the cholera research symposium. U.S. Public Health Serv. Publ. *1328*.

CHAMBERS, J.S. 1938. The Conquest of Cholera. Macmillan, New York.

FINKELSTEIN, R.A. 1973. Cholera. Crit. Rev. Microbiol. *2* (4) 553.

GANGAROSA, E.J. and MOSLEY, W.H. 1970. Asiatic cholera. *In* Tice's Practice of Medicine, Vol. 3. Harper and Row, Hagerstown, Md.

GANGAROSA, E.J. and MOSLEY, W.H. 1974. Epidemiologic surveillance of cholera. *In* Cholera. D. Barua and W. Burrows (Editors) W.B. Saunders Co., Philadelphia.

MAXEY, K.F. and ROSENAU, M.J. 1965. Preventive Medicine and Public Health, 9th Edition. P.E. Sartwell (Editor). Appleton-Century-Crofts, New York.

POLLITZER, R. 1959. Cholera. World Health Organization, Geneva.

SNOW, J. 1936. On Cholera. Commonwealth Fund, New York.

TOPLEY, W.W.C. and WILSON, G.S. 1975. The Principles of Bacteriology and Immunology, 6th Edition. Williams & Wilkins Co., Baltimore.

9

Clostridium perfringens Food Poisoning

Some cooks falsely believe that refrigerating hot foods, such as meats or fowl, too soon after they have been cooked, causes them to turn "sour." Then there are those who feel that hot food placed in the refrigerator will cause the motor to overwork and considerably increase their monthly utility bill. They will therefore permit such hot foods to cool slowly at room temperature, sometimes for several hours, before they decide to refrigerate them. Such conditions are most favorable for the growth and multiplication of Type C *Clostridium perfringens (C. welchii)*, a ubiquitous bacillus present on most raw meats and capable of causing a form of gastroenteritis.

The heat during cooking is believed to "activate" the spores produced by *C. perfringens*. The spores are heat resistant and capable of surviving boiling for 1 hr or longer. During cooling, the spores germinate promptly into vegetative cells that multiply actively, as *C. perfringens* grows well in temperatures up to 50°C, and best between 43° and 47°C.

Characteristics

C. perfringens is a Gram-positive, short, plump, rod-shaped, sporeforming bacillus, occurring singly or in pairs. It is capsulated and nonmotile. It is believed that, like *Staphylococcus*, it is capable of producing a heat resistant toxin in food before it is eaten, which may cause gastroenteritis. Another view is that an endotoxin is formed in the intestines by the dead bacilli after the contaminated food is ingested. Although *C. perfringens* is part of the normal flora of the intestinal tract of humans and animals, illness will result if it is further introduced into the intestines in exceedingly large numbers (millions per gram). It is also found in soil.

The incubation period of clostridial food poisoning is 8 to 22 hr, usually 10 to 12 hr. Illness lasting 24 hr or less consists of a mild form of gastroenteritis with sudden onset, nausea, intestinal cramps, and a pronounced diarrhea. Diagnosis is made by finding excessively large numbers of *C. perfringens* in suspected food as well as in the patient's feces.

Anaerobic conditions are necessary for the growth and multiplication of *C. perfringens*. Such conditions are provided by the mass of a roast, ham, stew, or stuffed fowl that is being cooked. It must also be remembered that cooking drives off the oxygen from the food, making it a good medium for the growth of the organism.

Outbreaks of gastroenteritis caused by *C. perfringens* have been reported after eating boiled and rolled meats, meat pies, creamed chicken, chicken croquettes, soups, and gravies at cafeterias or dining clubs. A common practice is for institutions, restaurants, and caterers to precook meats and fowl on the day previous to serving. They are then stored and subjected to various degrees of refrigeration until being reheated and served on the following day. It is during the slicing, reheating, and exposure of the meats that conditions favorable for the generation of illness occur.

Prevention and Control

It is almost impossible to prevent the contamination of meats and poultry with *C. perfringens* spores. However, it is possible to control the cooking and storage of such foods so as to prevent or retard the growth of the microorganism.

C. perfringens can grow at temperatures well below that of the average room, growth being prevented only at 15°C or below, and its spores can survive heat for 1 hr or longer in a closed steam kettle. Therefore, it is important to take preventive steps such as: (1) all meat dishes should be served hot as soon as they are cooked; (2) cooked foods should be cooled rapidly and adequately refrigerated until served; (3) reheating of stored food before serving should be rapid; for example, sliced meat should be heated quickly in its gravy.

McClung pointed out in 1945 that routine bacteriological examinations of food samples involved in food poisoning outbreaks did not include procedures that would reveal the presence of *C. perfringens*. He therefore suggested that in the future those who are investigating food outbreaks include the inoculation of suitable anaerobic media to determine whether *C. perfringens* is present in the suspected food in sufficiently large numbers to be responsible for the illness. Fecal specimens should be similarly examined. This is now routinely done.

REFERENCES

ANGELOTTI, R., HALL, N.E., FOSTER, M.J. and LEWIS, K.H. 1962. Quantitation of *Clostridium perfringens* in foods. Appl. Microbiol. *10*, 193.

BROWN, A.S., LYNCH, G., LEONARD, A.R. and STAFFORD, G. 1962. A clostridial or enterococcal food poisoning outbreak. Public Health Rep. *77*, 533.

HALL, N.E., ANGELOTTI, R., LEWIS, K.H. and FOSTER, H.J. 1963. The characteristics of *Clostridium perfringens* associated with food and foodborne diseases. J. Bacteriol. *85*, 1094.

HAUSCHILD, A.H.W. 1971. *Clostridium perfringens* enterotoxin. J. Milk Food Technol. *34*, 596.

HOBBS, B.C. 1960. Staphylococcal and *Clostridium welchii* food poisoning. J. R. Soc. Health *80*, 267.

HOBBS, B.C. *et al.* 1953. *Clostridium welchii* food poisoning. J. Hyg. *51*, 75.

LABBE, R.G. and DUNCAN, C.L. 1977. Spore coat protein and enterotoxin synthesis of *Clostridium perfringens*. J. Bacteriol. *131*, 713.

McCLUNG, L.S. 1976. Personal correspondence. Indiana Univ., Bloomington.

SPECK, M.L. 1976. Compendium of Methods for the Microbiological Examination of Foods. American Public Health Association, Washington, D.C.

STRONG, D.H., CANADA, J.J. and GRIFFITH, B.B. 1963. Incidence of *Clostridium perfringens* in American foods. Appl. Microbiol. *11*, 42.

10

Escherichia coli Diarrhea

Characteristics

Occasionally persons visiting one of the Latin American countries south of our border and partaking of their food and water come down with what is known as "traveler's diarrhea," referred to by the natives as "turista," and as "Montezuma's revenge" by travelers familiar with Mexican history. The illness, which lasts from 1 to 3 days, is characterized by severe diarrhea, abdominal pain, nausea, vomiting, and occasional fever.

This condition is brought about by 1 of the enteropathogenic forms of *Escherichia coli*, of which there are 2 types: (1) the invasive strain that attacks the colon causing symptoms similar to those of shigellosis, and (2) the enterotoxic strain with cholera-like symptoms with profuse watery stools, prostration, and dehydration. The latter produces toxins, some being thermostable and others thermolabile.

Sources of Infection

As in the case of brucellosis (see Chapter 11), meat-packing workers are exposed to these strains of *E. coli* that are a natural part of the flora of cattle and swine. Workers have been demonstrated to have serologic evidence of infection with the enterotoxic strains.

Foodborne and waterborne outbreaks of enteropathogenic *E. coli* diarrhea occur in communities with inadequate sanitation through fecal contamination of food or water. However, the more serious aspect of this problem, because of its potentially high fatality rate (up to 40%), is the occurrence of outbreaks of diarrhea in hospital newborn nurseries. Infants, particularly prematures, appear to be most susceptable to infection. Transmission of infection from one colonized infant with diarrhea to another in the nursery may occur because of inadequate sanitary conditions within the nursery, or poor handwashing of persons caring for

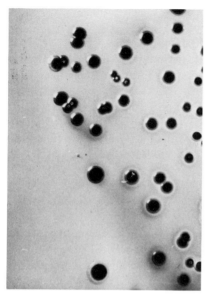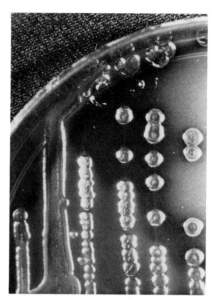

Courtesy of Elliot Scientific Corp. and Abbott Laboratories

FIG. 10.1. *ESCHERICHIA COLI*
LEFT—Culture on EMB agar.
RIGHT—Culture on Endo agar with positive lactose fermentation.

the infants, or by contaminated formulas. It may also be spread to infants by nursery personnel, who may be healthy carriers of the pathogenic *E. coli* organism, by faulty personal toilet hygiene. Illness of the infant occurs within 12 to 72 hr after infection.

Diagnosis and Treatment

Diagnosis is made by the isolation of pathogenic strains of *E. coli* from the patient's feces. The Sereny test (instillation in guinea pig's eye) will indicate invasiveness if keratoconjunctivitis results. Serotypes may be identified by serologic tests.

There is no specific treatment for enteropathogenic *E. coli* infection. Fluids and electrolyte fluids by mouth or intravenously are recommended. To relieve the diarrhea, nonabsorbable antibiotics may be used.

Prevention

Preventive measures are similar to those for typhoid fever and other diseases spread by the fecal-oral route. The prevention of outbreaks in hospital nurseries depends on:

(1) Scrupulous cleanliness of nursery.
(2) Proper handwashing practice of personnel.
(3) Aseptic formula preparation with periodic bacteriologic sampling.
(4) Separation of newborns and premature infants, each with its own personnel.
(5) Isolation of any infant with diarrhea and quarantine of new admissions.
(6) Infants born each day should be kept in separate area of nursery.
(7) Keep daily records of number and consistency of stools of each infant.

Control

If 2 or more cases of diarrhea occur in the nursery, notify the Department of Health and promptly isolate each infant. Cease admitting new babies to the nursery and discharge infected infants when possible. Separate medical and nursing personnel should be provided for the babies exposed in the contaminated nursery. Observe contacts in the nursery for at least 2 weeks after the last case has been discharged. Services may be resumed after all contact babies have been discharged and the nursery has been thoroughly cleansed and disinfected.

The following steps to be followed in conducting an epidemiologic investigation of an outbreak of diarrhea in a hospital nursery are outlined in *Communicable Diseases in Man, 12th Edition*, page 101 (Benenson 1975):

(a) Conduct an investigation into the distribution of cases by time, place, and person and exposure to risk factors to determine how transmission is occurring.
(b) Assume adequate treatment of missed cases by follow-up examination of all infants discharged from hospital during the two weeks preceding the first recognized case.
(c) Examine mothers and maternity service personnel for early signs of illness.
(d) Bacteriologic survey of ill and well infants is an important means of defining high risk areas and discovering reservoirs; also finding the suspect serotype in higher frequency among ill persons than among well ones helps establish its pathogenicity.
(e) Survey hospital for unsanitary conditions.
(f) Investigation of preparation of feeding formulae.
(g) Inquire into techniques of aseptic nursing of infants and changing diapers and other clothing. Chemoprophylaxis for contacts should be approached with caution but may have some value.

A report of such an investigation is given below in order to demonstrate how such steps may be put into practice. Although *E. coli* was isolated from the infants with diarrhea, determination of the serotype could not be made at that time.

OUTBREAK OF DIARRHEA OF NEWBORN AT MEADOWBROOK HOSPITAL, EAST MEADOW, N.Y.

The author received a telephone call at 2:30 P.M. on Sunday, July 17th from Dr. R.R., resident, Pediatric Services, Meadowbrook Hospital, that diarrhea had occurred among 7 newborns in the nursery.

Cases

A prompt visit to Meadowbrook Hospital revealed that the first watery stool was noted on July 16 at 2:00 P.M. The first baby involved (Baby A) was born on July 11 and was breast-fed, receiving some supplementary feeding. It had 3 more liquid stools on July 16, 2 of which were explosive in character. At 5:00 P.M., 3 other babies (Babies C, D, and E) had diarrhea. On the following day 2 more newborns (Babies B and F) and a month-old baby (Baby G), awaiting placement in a foster home, had watery stools. Two additional babies with diarrhea stools were subsequently reported on July 19 at 5:00 P.M. (Baby H) and on July 20 at 10:00 A.M. (Baby J). This made a total of 9 cases (Table 10.1).

Illness

Illness of the babies was mild. At no time was dehydration noted. The infants took their feedings and had no signs or symptoms other than diarrhea. The number of watery stools per day per infant varied, 4 being the highest daily number (Baby A). The others had from 2 to 3 such stools for 1 to 3 days (Table 10.1).

Nurseries

The infants were kept in 4 nurseries arranged in 2 sets of interconnecting pairs separated by an accessory room (Fig. 10.2).

Nursery 1 was used to keep babies born at the hospital and awaiting placement in foster homes. Their ages were from 1 to 4 months. Nursery 2 was used for neonates for the first 24 hr after which they were moved to nurseries 3 and 4. At the time of the outbreak there were 6 infants in nursery 1, none in nursery 2, 8 in nursery 3, and 9 in nursery 4, making a total of 23 infants. When the investigation was started on July 17, 1 infant from nursery 1, 3 from nursery 3, and 3 from nursery 4 were involved (see Table 10.2).

TABLE 10.1. DIARRHEA OF NEWBORN IN NURSERIES AT MEADOWBROOK HOSPITAL—JULY 16 TO JULY 20, 1955

Infant	Sex	Date of Birth	Nursery Number	Feeding Breast	Feeding Formula	Onset Date	Onset Time	7-16	7-17	7-18	7-19	7-20	Date of Discharge	Comments
A	F	7-11-55	4	X		7-16	2 P.M.	4	3	—	—	—	7-17	Omphalitis diagnosed 7-16 A.M.
B	M	7-14-55	3	X		7-17	9 P.M.	3	3	2	1		7-22	Developed eye infection 7-17
C	F	7-12-55	3		X	7-16	5 P.M.	1	3	1	—	—	7-18	
D	F	7-14-55	4		X	7-16	5 P.M.	1	2	1	—	—	7-18	
E	F	7-14-55	4		X	7-16	5 P.M.	1	2	1	—	—	7-18	
F	F	7-13-55	3		X	7-17	10 A.M.		3	2	1	1	7-20	
G	M	6-19-55	1		X	7-17	1:30 P.M.		1	2	1	—	—	Boarder transferred to Pediatric Ward 7-20
H	M	7-15-55	3		X	7-19	5 P.M.				1	2	7-20	
J	F	1-17-55	2		X	7-20	10 A.M.					2	7-21	

Number of Watery Stools (columns 7-16 through 7-20)

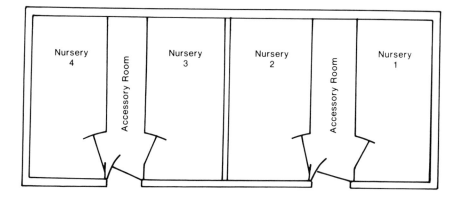

FIG. 10.2. NEWBORN NURSERIES AT MEADOWBROOK HOSPITAL

TABLE 10.2. CENSUS AND CASES OF DIARRHEA IN NURSERIES

Nursery Number	Census	Cases
1	6	1
2	0	0
3	8	3
4	9	3
Total	23	7

Baby B on July 17 developed an infection of the left eye. Laboratory examination revealed that the infection was caused by beta streptococci.

Control Measures at the Time of the Investigation

The 7 infants with diarrhea were transferred to an isolation nursery with a special nurse in charge of their care. Nurseries 3 and 4 were kept as "observation" nurseries, the exposed infants being quarantined there—the boarders in nursery 3 and the newborn infants in nursery 4.

New admissions were to be made only into nursery 2 which had had no illness and was considered "clean." Nursery 1 was to be scrubbed and aired and to remain unused for 2 days. It was recommended that the babies be discharged to their homes as expeditiously as possible where they would be followed up by a visit of the public health nurses. However, when on July 20 one of the newborns in the alleged "clean" nursery 2 was reported to have an explosive watery stool, it was decided to institute more drastic control measures and to stop all new admissions into the contaminated nurseries.

The choice was presented to the acting superintendent of the hospital of either closing the delivery room and nurseries to all new admissions or of opening a pair of never previously used nurseries located on the same floor but some distance from the contaminated ones for the admission of newborns from that time on. The latter course was chosen. The babies in nurseries 2, 3, and 4 were discharged to their homes within a few days, after which the nurseries were given a thorough scrubbing.

As no further diarrhea occurred, all restrictions were removed on July 25 and permission was granted to resume admissions into the 4 regular nurseries.

Laboratory Examinations

Examinations of stools of the infants with diarrhea made at the laboratories of Meadowbrook Hospital and the Nassau County Department of Health revealed a variety of microorganisms: *Escherichia coli, Enterobacter aerogenes*, a member of the *Proteus* group, alpha and beta streptococci, *Staphylococcus albus* and *S. aureus*, and diphtheroids. *E. coli* was isolated in large numbers.

The Meadowbrook Hospital laboratory also isolated *Branhamella catarrhalis*, beta *Streptococcus*, and *Staphylococcus albus* from the nose and throat of the infants.

Treatment

The infants with diarrhea received therapeutic doses of kaopectin with neomycin. The exposed infants received similar medication prophylactically.

Conference with Hospital Administrators and Others

Several conferences were held with various members of the hospital administrative, medical, and nursing staffs. On July 18 the author met with the acting superintendent of the hospital, the medical resident in charge of newborn nursery service, and the attending physicians on nursery service in order to discuss control measures. A hospital-consultant-public health nurse also held a conference on that day with various members of the hospital nursing staff at which time she reviewed: (1) the physical facilities of the nursery; (2) the preparation, processing, and storage of the formulas; (3) newborn techniques and practices; (4) the activities of the nursing personnel assigned to the newborn nursery; and (5) other pertinent data necessary in order to complete the questionnaire used in making yearly inspections of hospitals. She reviewed Chapter II,

Regulation 35, of the New York State Sanitary Code [N.Y. State Health Counc. (undated)] with the group and pointed out several violations, the major ones being the boarding of infants over 28 days in the newborn nursery, and the interflow of nurses among the nurseries due to the shortage of the nursing staff. She also inspected the formula room but found only a minor violation—the formula thermometer was not self-registering.

After another conference with representatives of the hospital and the New York State Department of Health, Division of Child Health, it was decided to insist that the delivery room and nursery section be closed to new admissions and that the new set of nurseries not located within the newborn service be placed in operation.

Follow-up

Following the initial investigation a follow-up study was made. Daily contact was kept up with the hospital administrator and the medical resident in order to obtain information regarding the progress of the infants with diarrhea, the exposed babies in the observation nurseries, and the newborn infants in the fresh "clean" nurseries.

The public health consultant nurse visited the newborn nursery service on July 22 to inspect the "clean" nurseries and to check upon their servicing.

Public health nurses were requested to visit the homes of 8 of the infants who had had diarrhea while at the hospital. The ninth baby remained in the hospital still awaiting adoption or placement in a home. Similar visits were made to the homes of 19 other infants born at the hospital and discharged from July 13 to July 20 in a quest for missed cases of diarrhea. All were found to be in good health.

Probable Causes of Outbreak

No definite conclusion can be made as to the cause of the outbreak of diarrhea among the infants. There were uncovered during the investigation, however, the following 4 conditions, any of which could have been a factor:

(1) Infection of umbilicus: The first infant to develop diarrhea (Baby A) was discovered on the morning of July 16 to have an infected umbilicus with a purulent exudate. The baby was not removed from nursery 4 until after 6 other infants had developed diarrhea on the following day. On culture of the pus, *Escherichia coli* and *Staphylococcus aureus* were isolated. The same microorganisms were found in the stools of 5 infants with diarrhea.

(2) Nursing baby's mother with sore throat: A post-partum patient who was breast-feeding her infant had had a sore throat and fever since July 15. Culture of her throat revealed *Branhamella catarrhalis* and alpha and beta streptococci. Her baby was kept in nursery 4 where the outbreak initiated. Although this infant had no diarrhea, it could have introduced the infection from its mother into the nursery.

(3) Delivery room nurse with sore throat: It was learned that one of the nurses on service in the delivery room had had a sore throat for several days. She is alleged to have handled some of the infants in the nursery on the morning of July 16. *Branhamella catarrhalis* and alpha streptococci were isolated from her throat on culture.

(4) Delivery room nurse with attack of gastroenteritis: On July 10 an outbreak of food poisoning characterized by nausea, vomiting, abdominal cramps, and diarrhea occured in 16 out of 222 employees on the night shift of Meadowbrook Hospital 2 to 4 hr after eating their midnight dinner. It is believed that the illness was caused by a tray full of roast chicken which was left out of the refrigerator for about 5 hr. One of the persons involved was one of the night nurses on service in the delivery room. It was learned that she assisted in the delivery of Baby A on the night of July 11 and handled it immediately after birth. It should be remembered that Baby A was the first infant to have diarrhea on July 16.

Summary

An outbreak of diarrhea occurred in the well-baby nursery at Meadowbrook Hospital. A total of 9 infants had from 2 to 4 watery stools daily between July 16 and July 20. Illness was mild and all recovered within 3 to 5 days. An investigation was made on July 17 and prompt control measures instituted. All discharged infants were followed up by public health nurses. Several adverse conditions were found, one or more of which could have been responsible for the outbreak.

REFERENCES

BENENSON, A.S. 1975. Control of Communicable Diseases in Man, 12th Edition. American Public Health Association, Washington, D.C.

COMMUNICABLE DIS. CENT. 1976. Diarrheal illness on a cruise ship by enterotoxigenic *Escherichia coli*. Morbidity Mortality *25*, 229.

DuPONT, H.D. *et al.* 1977. Pathogenesis of *Escherichia coli* diarrhea. N. Engl. J. Med. *285*, 1.

GORBACK, S.L. and KHURANA, C.M. 1972. Toxigenic *Escherichia coli*. A cause of infantile diarrhea in Chicago. N. Engl. J. Med. *287*, 791.

KLUPSTEIN, F.A., ENGERT, R.F. and SHORT, H.B. 1977. Relative enterotoxigenicity of coliform bacteria. J. Infect. Dis. *136*, 205.

MEHLMAN, I.J. *et al.* 1977. Methodology for recognition of invasive potential of *Escherichia coli*. J. Assoc. Off. Anal. Chem. *60*, 546.

MERSON, M.H. *et al.* 1975. Travelers' diarrhea in Mexico: A prospective study. 16th Inter-sci. Conf. Antimicrobial Agents Chemotherapy. Am. Soc. Microbiol., Sept. 24–26, 1975. Washington, D.C.

NETER, E. 1975. Enteropathogenicity of *Escherichia coli*. Am. J. Dis. Child. *129*, 666.

N.Y. STATE HEALTH COUNC. (Undated). New Born Nurseries. Chapter 2. N.Y. State Sanitary Code, Albany, Reg. *35*.

RUDOY, R.C. and NELSON, J.D. 1975. Enteroinvasive and enterotoxigenic *Escherichia coli*. Am. J. Dis. Child. *129*, 668.

SACK, R.B. 1975. Human diarrheal disease caused by enterotoxigenic *Escherichia coli*. Annu. Rev. Microbiol. *29*, 335.

SACK, R.B. *et al.* 1975. Enterotoxigenic *Escherichia coli*-associated diarrheal disease in Apache children. N. Engl. J. Med. *292*, 1041.

SACK, R.B. *et al.* 1977. Enterotoxigenic *Escherichia coli* isolated from food. J. Infect. Dis. *135*, 313.

WALLACE, R.B. and DONTA, S.T. 1978. Antibody to *Escherichia coli* enterotoxin in meat-packing workers. Am. J. Public Health *68*, 68.

11

Brucellosis

Mandatory pasteurization of commercially sold milk and milk products (cream, butter, and cheese) and the progressive control of infection among animals, particularly cattle, through testing and immunization against Bang's disease, have resulted in a marked decline of human brucellosis in the United States. However, cases are still encountered in some midwestern states, in Mexico, South America, and in the Mediterranean countries of Europe, Africa, and Asia.

Sources of Infection

For many years, brucellosis, also known as undulant fever, has been considered to be an occupational disease of persons working with infected domestic animals such as cattle, sheep, goats, swine, and horses. Veterinary surgeons, farm workers, butchers, and packing-house employees are at special risk. Cows become infected by ingesting *Brucella* organisms and developing placentitis followed by abortion. The fetus, placenta, and discharges are loaded with viable bacilli, infecting persons with abrasions on their hands who handle these tissues.

As infection in the cow is often located in the udder, *Brucella* bacilli are constantly or intermittently excreted in the milk. Humans who consume such milk or any of its products without their having been pasteurized or boiled invariably acquire the disease.

Characteristics

Recognition of brucellosis is often difficult because of its diverse symptoms, variable course, and absence of distinguishing features. It is a debilitating systemic disease. Its onset may be sudden or insidious as its incubation period is from 5 to 21 days. Its most characteristic symptom is fever of various duration that may be continuous, intermittent, or irregular, low in the morning and rising in the afternoon and evening.

Patients also complain of weakness, headache, anorexia, chills, sweating, generalized aches, arthralgia (joint pains), and depression. Splenomegaly and lymphadenopathy are often noted. The duration of the disease may be several days or it may become chronic, lasting for several years.

The infectious agents of brucellosis consist of several species of *Brucella*, the more common being: (1) *Brucella abortus*, spread by cattle and accounting for most human cases, is the least invasive infection; (2) *Brucella suis*, from hogs, although cattle and horses are also susceptible to its infection, is more virulent than *B. abortus*; (3) *Brucella melitensis*, from goats and sheep, more common in Mexico than in the United States, and causing the most severe illness as man appears to be most susceptible to it.

Following the introduction of the *Brucella* in the bloodstream through the abraded skin or the gastrointestinal tract, it localizes within 24 hr in the lymph nodes, liver, spleen, and bone marrow. In chronic cases there is formation of granulomas, necrosis, and casiation in these tissues that may persist for 20 to 25 years. If the disease is unrecognized and untreated, it may lead to such disabling conditions as spondylitis (inflammation of the vertebrae), meningitis, and subacute endocarditis.

Diagnosis

Definite diagnosis of brucellosis may be made by the positive isolation of *Brucella* bacilli on culture of blood, bone marrow, or other tissues early in the course of the disease. Agglutination tests with elevation of titer in repeated serum specimens is another diagnostic aid. A titer of 1 to 80 or below is seldom significant. However, a titer that is low early and rises later is strong evidence of active disease. Consideration should be given to the possibility of an anamnestic reaction as a high *Brucella* agglutination titer may be produced by tularemia, cholera, or vaccination against cholera.

A positive reaction with the *Brucella* skin test may be misleading as it merely indicates sensitivity to the *Brucella* antigen even though active infection is not present. This may occur because of previous asymptomatic infection with *Brucella*. A negative skin test will rule out infection but a positive reaction by itself is of little value in diagnosing brucellosis. Besides, the skin test may induce a rise in titer and confuse agglutination testing.

Prevention

Eradication of the disease in cattle is the only positive method that is likely to eliminate the danger of brucellosis to the public health. In endemic areas, immunization of calves is recommended. The testing of livestock for Bang's disease with segregation or slaughter of infected animals is necessary. Milk from cows, goats, or sheep should be pasteurized (or boiled). Farmers, butchers, and slaughterhouse workers should be made acquainted of the dangers of handling the meat or products of infected animals. Farmers and cattle breeders, in particular, should be instructed in the hazard of handling the fetus, placenta, and discharges of aborted animals.

Control

Reported cases and outbreaks should be promptly investigated for a common vehicle of infection (raw milk or animal contact). If raw milk is involved, its distribution should be stopped and pasteurization provided. Even if on investigating an outbreak it is learned that all the patients drank milk from a dairy that allegedly pasteurizes its milk, it is wise to check the pasteurization records at the dairy to determine whether there was a breakdown of the machinery at any time previous to the outbreak.

Treatment

Specific treatment for acute brucellosis is lacking. Bed rest with supportive treatment is extremely helpful. Symptoms may be allayed with tetracycline or its derivatives, 0.5 g 4 to 6 times daily for 3 weeks. In severe cases or if abscesses are present, streptomycin may be added. Corticosteroids should be administered to decrease systemic toxicity. The relapse rate is 5 to 20% depending on which species of *Brucella* is involved. Treatment should be resumed for a period of 10 days with larger doses if relapse occurs.

Investigations of Outbreaks

The findings in the investigations of a limited outbreak and of 2 individual cases of brucellosis that occurred locally are given as illustrations.

Familial Outbreak.—On investigating an outbreak in 4 members of a family, it was learned that the head of the household, a railroad employee, had decided in view of the high cost of milk to purchase a cow and do his own milking. He was able to pay a low price for her because she was "slightly sick" which he believed was due to improper feeding. It turned out on examination by the county veterinarian and on blood culture that the animal had Bang's disease and had not been previously tested or vaccinated. The milk had been consumed raw by the members of the family, all of whom developed brucellosis. It was a regrettable decision and a grievous bargain!

Imported Case.—A 53-year-old physician from Lima, Peru, was visiting the United States. Shortly before leaving Lima, he had stopped for several days at a coastal city where he had milk and other dairy products. He subsequently learned that there was an epidemic of brucellosis in that city. While in Nassau County, he developed fever, chills, and severe headaches. Three days after onset, he vomited blood and was admitted to a local hospital where an organism isolated on blood culture was identified by the laboratory of the New York State Department of Health as *Brucella melitensis*. Incidentally, a gastrointestinal X-ray examination revealed that the patient had a duodenal ulcer that accounted for the hemoptysis.

Laboratory Infection.—Early in June, a 48-year-old male, employed as a microbiologist at the laboratory at the North Shore Hospital located in Manhasset, N.Y., developed headache and vague grippe-like symptoms. This was followed by intermittent fever, chills, malaise profuse sweating, and muscular aches. He was admitted to the hospital on August 13th where agglutination was obtained with *Brucella abortus* antigen in a titer of 320 dilution of his serum. Three weeks later the titer rose to 1280. On culture of his bone marrow and blood, *B. melitensis* was isolated. He was treated with streptomycin, 0.5 g twice a day for 7 days, and tetracycline, 500 mg 4 times a day. On questioning, he stated that in April and May he had examined specimens of lymph gland tissue, bone marrow, and blood from a patient suspected of having become infected with brucellosis while visiting Italy. He isolated *B. melitensis* from the specimens. In June he had transplanted the isolated microorganisms for further study. It appeared that contact with the *Brucella* organisms in the laboratory resulted in his infection.

REFERENCES

BENENSON, A.S. 1975. Communicable Diseases in Man, 12th Edition. American Public Health Association, Washington, D.C.

BRYAN, F.L. 1969. Infections due to miscellaneous microorganisms. *In* Foodborne Infections and Intoxications. H. Rieman (Editor). Academic Press, New York.

EISELL, C.W. 1950. Current problems in the diagnosis and treatment of brucellosis. Wis. Med. J. *49*, 201.

HARRIS, H.J. 1941. Brucellosis (Undulent Fever). Paul B. Hoeber, New York.

MINGLE, C.K. 1959. Progress report on cooperative state-federal brucellosis eradication program. U.S. Dep. Agric., Agric. Res. Serv., (Feb.).

WHITE, P.C., JR. *et al.* 1974. Brucellosis in a Virginia meat packing plant. Arch. Environ. Health *28*, 263.

W.H.O. 1959. Diseases common to man and other animals. Joint W.H.O./F.A.O. Tech. Rep. Ser. Expert Comm. Zoonosis *169*, 6.

12

Tularemia

The man who picks up his gun, whistles to his dog, and starts out for a day's hunt for wild rabbits, is, no doubt, fully aware of the dangers which may result from the careless handling of firearms. He may not, however, suspect that danger also lurks in the bodies of the apparently harmless little animals he is carrying home in his bag. The homemaker and the cook who dress or handle wild rabbits, and the trapper whose hands come in contact with the raw flesh and blood of the rodents whose pelts he is removing for the market, may be exposing themselves to a risk unknown to them.

The disease which man may acquire in his search for fun, food, and fur is known as tularemia. It causes prolonged morbidity and disability and has a case fatality rate of 5%. Cases have been reported in all states in the United States as well as in several foreign countries.

Characteristics

Tularemia is primarily an acute infectious disease of wild rodents which may result in an accidental infection of man. It is also known as rabbit fever and deerfly fever. The etiologic agent, previously called *Pasteurella tularensis*, because it causes pasteurellosis (hemorrhagic septicemia), is now referred to as *Francisella tularensis.*

The name *Francisella tularensis* that has been given to the infective agent is in honor of Dr. Edward Francis who named the disease after Tulare County in California where it was first discovered and traced to wild rabbits.

Francisella tularensis is pleomorphic or variable in form. Most often it is bacillary, but coccoid or bipolar forms are noted. It is Gram-negative, aerobic, nonmotile, and nonspore-bearing. It is readily destroyed by ordinary disinfectants and by temperatures above 56°C.

Sources of Infection

Infected wild rabbits and wild hares are the direct cause of over 90% of human cases in the United States. A number of other wild animals susceptible to the disease and capable of transmitting it to man are the ground and tree squirrel, woodchuck, opossum, raccoon, skunk, beaver, fox, shrew, chipmunk, guinea pig, deer, bull snake, and various types of rats and mice. Among birds, infection has been reported in grouse, quail, sage hen, owl, and gull. The domestic dog, cat, sheep, and calf have also been found infected.

The disease is transmitted to animals principally by the bite of infected blood-sucking arachnida or insects, such as the tick, deerfly, rat flea, squirrel flea, rabbit tick, louse, and flea. The main and permanent reservoir of infection is the wood tick, *Dermacentor andersoni*, and the dog tick, *Dermacentor variabolis*, which are capable of transmitting the infection through eggs on to successive generations. The rabbit tick, *Haemaphysalis leporis-palustris*, which rarely bites man but transmits infection from rabbit to rabbit, is also an important vector. Occasionally animals contract the disease by eating the carcass of another infected animal.

Tularemia may be transmitted to humans in one of several ways: (1) inoculation through broken skin of the hands with the blood or the tissues of infected rabbits or hares or other edible animals while skinning or dressing them; (2) directly by the bite of arthropods or insects such as infected ticks or deerflies; (3) ingestion of insufficiently cooked meat of infected rabbit or hare; (4) drinking contaminated water; (5) inhalation of dust from contaminated soil or hay; (6) laboratory infection.

Persons whose occupations or recreational inclinations expose them to contact with animals and insects have a high infection rate. Hunters, market people, butchers, cooks, and homemakers who skin and dress wild rabbits with bare hands become ill as the result of contact with the blood, liver, spleen, or bone marrow of an infected animal. In most instances, the point of entry of the organism is a wound of the hand inflicted shortly before by barbed wire, nail, thorn, or burr, or at the time of contact by a knife or bone fragment.

Campers, woodsmen, and foresters are exposed to bites from infected ticks or deerflies. Sheep shearers and herders acquire the disease through contact with wood ticks and their feces located on the wool of sheep.

Improperly cooked infected wild rabbit meat may also cause illness. Infection of 43 persons resulting from drinking contaminated water was observed in Russia in 1935. Incidental to studies of epizootic tularemia in beavers, Public Health Service workers found that the water in 3 Montana streams was contaminated with *F. tularensis*.

Clinical Diagnosis

Tularemia may assume several clinical forms, the most common being the ulceroglandular type. After an incubation period of 2 to 4 days after contact, the onset of illness comes on suddenly with chills, fever, backache, sweats, vomiting, and body aches. A local lesion that soon ulcerates appears on the abraded skin of the finger or at the site of the insect bite, and lymph nodes that drain the area become tender and indurated.

People who eat inadequately cooked infected rabbit meat or drink contaminated water develop the typhoid type of infection in which the general symptoms are present but neither the initial lesion nor the bubo (inflamed lymph gland) occur. Other forms are: the glandular type with the absence of the primary lesion but the constitutional symptoms and the bubo present; the oculoglandular type in which the hand carries the infection from the flesh of the infected animal to the eye, causing a severe inflammatory reaction; and the pulmonary type, resulting in pneumonia with pleural effusion with a high fatality rate.

In the majority of cases, tularemia is easily diagnosed. A careful history will often uncover information regarding the handling, skinning, cleaning, or eating of wild rabbit or another form of wildlife, or of the bite of a tick or insect. The presence of the initial ulceration and the bubo plus the general sepsis make the diagnosis obvious.

Clinical diagnosis is confirmed by means of the agglutination reaction and by isolation of the causative microorganism through animal inoculation and cultures. Agglutinins appear in the blood during the second week of illness and may reach a titer of 1 to 1280 within the third week. These agglutinins may persist for many years after recovery. Blood serum from a patient with tularemia may cross-agglutinate *Brucella abortus* and *Brucella melitensis* organisms, the causative agents of undulant and Malta fever.

Guinea pig or rabbit inoculation with the exudate from the initial lesion or from the bubo, or with blood of the patient obtained during the septicemic stage, offers additional diagnostic aid.

The intradermal test, which consists of the injection of 0.01 ml of tularemia antigen, if performed on the fourth day of illness, frequently gives a positive local reaction in 48 hr. It is not considered altogether reliable, however.

Treatment

The drug of choice for the treatment of tularemia is streptomycin. If tetracycline or chloramphenicol is given, it should be continued until the temperature is normal for 4 or 5 days.

Prevention

The most practical means of preventing tularemia is avoidance of direct contact of the bare hands with infected wild animals. It is recommended that the following advice be made available to hunters, cooks, homemakers, and market people:

(1) The hunter should not kill or handle a wild rabbit or hare which is too sick to run or which is caught by a dog. According to Hendrickson (1937): "The sick animal (tularemic rabbit) doesn't raise the head, doesn't carry the front feet well, rubs the nose and front feet into the earth, lies in tremors, staggers along a few rods, and again lies in tremors."

(2) Rubber gloves should be worn when skinning and dressing wild rabbit. A person who has sores or cuts on his hands should not clean rabbits.

(3) Care should be taken not to puncture the gloves and injure the hands with a knife or bone fragments. If the skin is injured, the wound should be immediately washed with soap and water, after which an antiseptic solution should be applied to the injury. Rubber gloves should be washed with soap and water, and disinfected. Disposable gloves should be discarded.

(4) The liver, spleen, and lungs of the rabbit should be examined when the carcass is being dressed. The presence of small white spots may indicate that the animal has tularemia. Such an infected carcass should be burned or buried so as not to be eaten by a dog or cat.

(5) The liberal use of soap and water followed by disinfection of the hands is recommended in order to remove all rabbit blood from the hands. Even when only the fur is handled, the hands should be thoroughly washed.

(6) The hands of the rabbit handler should be kept away from the eyes.

(7) Wild rabbit meat should be thoroughly cooked from surface to center in order to destroy the organism causing tularemia as it will remain alive and virulent in the red juice of the bones of partly cooked game. Refrigeration does not kill the organisms, as rabbits kept constantly frozen at $-15°C$ may remain infective for $3\frac{1}{2}$ years.

(8) During the summer, hunters, trappers, campers, and woodsmen should wear tick-proof clothing, with trousers tucked into the shoes in order to avoid bites from infected ticks.

(9) Raw drinking water should be avoided in known infected areas.

(10) Laboratory workers have developed tularemia while doing autopsies on infected guinea pigs and rabbits or while handling infected ticks. A live vaccine obtainable from the National Communicable Disease Center, Atlanta, Ga., given intradermally by the multiple puncture method (as is used in smallpox vaccination) has proven effective in preventing laboratory infections.

REFERENCES

BENENSON, A.S. 1975. Control of Communicable Diseases in Man, 12th Edition. Am. Public Health Assoc., Washington, D.C.

BRYAN, F.L. 1969. Infections due to miscellaneous microorganisms. *In* Foodborne Infections and Intoxications. H. Riemann (Editor). Academic Press, New York.

FRANCIS, E. 1921. The occurrence of tularemia in nature as a disease of man. Public Health Rep. *36*, 1731.

FRANCIS, E. 1946. Personal correspondence. National Institutes of Health, October 1.

HENDRICKSON, G.O. 1937. Trans. 2nd North Am. Wild Life Conf., Am. Wild Life Inst.

MERCK AND CO. 1977. The Merck Manual of Diagnosis and Therapy, 13th Edition. Merck, Sharp and Dohme Research Laboratories, Division of Merck & Co., Rahway, N.J.

TARTAKOW, I.J. 1946. Tularemia in New York State. N.Y. State J. Med. *46*, 1329.

TARTAKOW, I.J. 1977. Casebook of a medical detective: A review of interesting cases. Nassau County Med. Cent. *4* (2) 65−73.

13

Leptospirosis

Leptospirosis, also known as Weil's disease, canicola fever, hemorrhagic jaundice, and swineherd's disease, may occur among swimmers exposed to waters contaminated with the urine of infected domestic or wild animals. It is also considered to be an occupational disease of individuals who come in direct contact with infected animals, such as veterinarians, farmers, animal husbandmen, and abbattoir workers, and may also attack persons who have contact with the urine of animals having the disease, such as rice and sugarcane field workers, sewer workers, employees in dog kennels, and dog owners.

Characteristics

The disease is caused by one of a number of serotypes of *Leptospira*, a finely coiled, spiral shaped, actively mobile bacterium. For many years strains of *Leptospira* have been compared and distinguished serologically by laboratories, especially by means of the agglutination reaction and cross-agglutination in absorption studies carried out with antisera prepared in rabbits. A number of serotypes of *Leptospira* have been recovered, among the most common in the United States being *Leptospira icterohaemorrhagiae, L. pomona, L. canicola,* and *L. autumnalis.* Many other serotypes have been recognized in various parts of the world.

According to *Bergey's Manual of Determinative Bacteriology, 8th Edition* (Buchanan and Gibbons 1974), the taxonomy or classification of the genus *Leptospira* is at the present time under consideration by the Subcommittee on Leptospira of the International Committee on Systematic Bacteriology. The subcommittee feels that there are not yet sufficient reliable taxonomic data for the circumscription of more than 1 species of *Leptospira.* It has therefore recommended that until further study only 1 species be recognized, namely *Leptospira enterrogans.*

Infection is characterized by fever and chills, headaches, malaise, vomiting, muscular pains, conjunctivitis, meningeal irritation, occasional jaundice, renal insufficiency, hemolytic anemia, and hemorrhages in skin and mucous membranes. The disease may manifest 3 phases: (1) bacteremia or septicemia which lasts 2 to 7 days; (2) icteric or toxic stage which begins on the 5th or 6th day; (3) convalescence or death. Illness lasts from several days to 3 weeks with relapses occurring in some instances. The fatality rate is low but may reach as high as 20% among elderly patients.

Leptospirosis occurs when the leptospirae penetrate a swimmer's or worker's abraded skin or mucous membranes, as well as by the ingestion of water polluted with urine from infected rats or dogs. Its incubation period is usually 10 days but may be from 4 to 20 days.

Sources of Infection

The reservoir of infection consists of a large number of animals, among them cattle, swine, dogs, deer, foxes, skunks, racoons, rats, and other rodents.

Although infected rats may appear anywhere, farmers may be exposed as well to infected domestic animals, hunters and trappers to wild animals, and city dwellers to dogs. Dogs may acquire canicola fever through their habit of licking urine and bringing their nose and tongue in contact with other dogs' genitals as well as through their mating act. Thus the virulent organisms penetrate the mucous membranes, enter the blood, and localize in the liver and the inner walls of the convoluted tubules of the kidneys where they multiply and are shed in the urine. Other possible routes of infection for dogs are contaminated water and food. Infected dog urine contains leptospira during illness and for a period of 4 to 6 months after recovery. Even the voided urine itself may reman infectious for days under favorable conditions, such as in neutral or slightly alkaline water at low temperatures. Transmission from dog to dog or dog to human may occur by contact with such infected urine.

Diagnosis

When examination of a patient discloses the following triad of clinical signs—conjunctivitis, aseptic meningitis, and albuminuria—the examiner should inquire as to the patient's occupation and/or contact with animals. If the reply is significant, then he should forward a sample of the patient's blood and urine to the laboratory for agglutination and complement fixation tests, culture of leptospirae, and guinea pig inoculation.

Prevention

In investigating an outbreak of leptospirosis, a search should be made for the source of infection, such as a pond used for swimming and occupational or home direct contact with animals.

The following preventive measures are recommended:

(1) Workers in hazardous occupations should be protected by boots and gloves.
(2) The public should be educated to avoid swimming or wading in potentially contaminated waters and should wear proper protection when work requires such exposure.
(3) Rat control in human habitations and the firing of cane fields before harvest.
(4) Sick domestic animals should be segregated in order to prevent contamination of living, working, and recreational areas.
(5) Vaccination of farm and pet animals.

Treatment

Although such antibiotics as penicillin, streptomycin, and tetracycline are leptospirocidal, they do not appear at all times to be of value in the treatment of human leptospirosis. They should be given early and in high dosage.

INVESTIGATION OF A CASE OF LEPTOSPIROSIS

The description of an investigation made by the senior author (I.J.T.) of a case of leptospirosis caused by the canicola serotype (canicola fever) follows. It illustrates the importance of inquiring into the patient's occupation; it describes the course of the disease and discusses the laboratory examination of the patient and of the animals suspected of being the source of infection.

History and Symptoms

A 16-year-old white male residing in Wantagh, N.Y., was suddenly taken ill on December 5, 1950, with chills and fever, anorexia, dizziness, frontal headache, and general malaise. This was shortly followed by muscular pains, abdominal cramps, nausea, vomiting, and diarrhea. The fever ran a relapsing course, rising on occasions to 39.4°C (103°F); the vomiting became more frequent and the headache more intense. On the eighth day of illness, the patient's mother noticed that his conjunctivae were markedly congested, and his eyes as well as his skin had taken on a yellowish tinge. He had several periods during which he was delirious and confused.

On December 25, the 20th day of illness, he developed rigidity of the neck. Diarrhea persisted to the extent that he had no control over his bowels. He was admitted to Meadowbrook Hospital, Hempstead, N.Y., on the following day with tentative diagnosis of nonparalytic poliomyelitis.

His past history revealed that he had had measles, mumps, chickenpox, and whooping cough during childhood. He had sustained a back injury following a fall at the age of 5 which had resulted in a mild kyphosis and scoliosis. He had been living at home with his parents and 4 siblings, none of whom had any acute illness.

Workplace

The patient had been employed for the past 6 months at the Bide-A-Wee Home for Friendless Animals located in Wantagh, N.Y. This is a philanthropic organization which houses, treats, and places approximately 3000 dogs yearly and is able to accommodate about 300 dogs at a time. During the first month of his employment he was assigned to the dog cemetery where he handled and buried the bodies of dogs. The next 2 months were spent in the "puppy house" where he fed the young dogs and kept their cages clean. During the past 3 months he had worked in the observation kennels where all newly acquired dogs are quarantined and sick dogs are isolated. His duties consisted of cleaning the kennels, cages, and runs, and of emptying, cleaning, and refilling the drinking troughs. The dogs habitually urinated into the troughs and it was necessary for him to move and handle these receptacles. His hands came in contact daily with the urine polluted water.

Admission to Hospital

On admission to the hospital his temperature was 38.3°C (101°F), pulse rate 80, and respiration rate 20 per min. He had signs of moderate meningeal irritation manifested as nuchal rigidity, diarrhea with fecal incontinence, listlessness, and disorientation. He had hallucinations, and it became necessary shortly after admission to restrain him as he became markedly agitated and fought his nurses and attendants. During lucid moments he complained of fever, headache, and abdominal cramps. No impairment of muscular function was observed.

Laboratory Findings

Spinal tap performed on December 26, the day of admission, produced clear cerebrospinal fluid under apparently normal pressure in which no white blood cells were seen but which contained 59 mg % of protein.

Laboratory findings on the following day included hemoglobin 12.5 g %, white blood cells 3800/mm³, with 62% polymorphonuclear leukocytes, 36% lymphocytes, and 2% monocytes. Albumin (2 plus), coarsely granular casts, and red blood cells were found in the urine. No bacteria incitant of enteric disease were isolated on culture of the stool. Blood nonprotein nitrogen was 43 mg % and blood sugar 105 mg %. The Kahn reaction on the blood serum was negative.

On December 29 urinanalysis again revealed albumin, hyaline casts, pus cells, and erythrocytes. On differential white blood cell count there was reported 6300 leucocytes with 70% polymorphonuclear cells, 28% lymphocytes, and 2% monocytes. Blood serum specimens examined both at the hospital laboratory and the Division of Laboratories and Research, New York State Department of Health, gave no sufficient agglutination with *S. typhosa* (O and H), *S. paratyphosa* (A and B), *Brucella abortus*, *Francisella tularensis*, and *Proteus X* strains.

In view of the occupational history of the patient, the possibility of leptospirosis was considered. Blood specimens were submitted to the Division of Laboratories and Research, New York State Department of Health, and agglutination reaction was reported with the serotype *Leptospira canicola* in increasing dilutions of the serum on the following dates:

> 1:1000 dilution on December 29, 1950
> 1:2000 dilution on January 8, 1951
> 1:4000 dilution on February 23, 1951
> 1:4000 dilution on March 30, 1951

No agglutination with serotype *Leptospira icterohaemorrhagiae* was obtained at any time. No *Leptospira* were recovered on guinea pig inoculation from a sample of urine examined on January 8.

Treatment

Although large quantities of valuable antibiotics are wasted daily through their indiscriminate administration in febrile diseases before diagnosis is made and the etiological agent is determined, there are occasions when, to the good fortune of the patient, the early empirical use of a certain antibiotic proves to be the therapeutic measure of choice. In this instance, penicillin therapy was started on the day of admission to the hospital. Intramuscular injection of 300,000 units was given every 8 hr for 7 days until 20 doses or a total of 6 million units had been given. Improvement was noted on the third day of treatment and the patient became afebrile on the fourth day. His further progress was uneventful and he was discharged from the hospital on January 2, 1951, the 28th day of illness.

Investigation of Possible Sources of Infection

With the cooperation of the veterinarians of the Nassau County Department of Health, blood specimens were secured on January 10, 1951,
from the random sample of 11 apparently well dogs, and urine specimens on January 23 from 5 dogs at the kennel. The blood samples were
delivered promptly to the Division of Laboratories and Research, Nassau
County Department of Health, where they were centrifuged in order to
prevent hemolysis, and the serum was sent to the State Department of
Health for examination. The serum of 4 of the dogs gave no significant
agglutination with either serotype *L. canicola* or *L. icterohaemorrhagiae.*
Agglutination with *L. canicola* occurred in a 1:50 dilution with 2 dog
sera, in a 1:100 dilution with 1 serum, and in a 1:500 dilution with 4 dog
sera. Significant agglutination was not obtained with *L. icterohaemorrhagiae* in any of the animal sera. The urine samples were injected into
guinea pigs which were sent to the State Department of Health for study,
but no evidence of infection with leptospirosis could be demonstrated in
these animals.

Conclusion

The history of contact with diseased dogs, the clinical course of the
patient's illness, and the serological evidence of acute infection of the
patient and latent infection in 45% of a random sample of dogs at the
patient's place of employment justifies the diagnosis of canicola fever.

Establishing a Diagnosis

As leptospirosis canicola may be and most probably is easily confused
with influenza, undulant fever, meningitis, or poliomyelitis, the assistance of the laboratory is indispensible in establishing the diagnosis. It is
unfortunate, however, that many laboratories are not equipped to properly carry out the required examinations.

The type of examination which should be performed depends upon the
stage of the disease. During the first week or in the septicemic stage,
leptospirae may be found in the blood and often in the spinal fluid. These
may be demonstrated by darkfield microscopic examination, culture
media, and animal inoculation. Leptospirae usually appear in the urine
during the second week of illness.

Difficulty is often encountered in their isolation from the urine as well
as the blood. The organism is destroyed by acid urine, and the usual
laboratory animal, such as the guinea pig, rat, and mouse, is resistant to
infection with *L. canicola*. The animal which has been found to be most
susceptible to intraperitoneal injection with *L. canicola* is the 3- to
4-week-old hamster.

After 12 to 14 days following onset, sufficient agglutinins appear in the patient's serum to produce a significant agglutination reaction (dilution of 1:100 or greater). The maximum titer is reached within 3 to 4 weeks and reaction is maintained for months or years after recovery.

Serological tests by various investigators have shown that 11 to 38% of dogs in various parts of this country show residuals of latent infection with leptospirae. It has been demonstrated that about 90% of the cases of canine leptospirosis are caused by *L. canicola*, and 10% by *L. icterohaemorrhagiae*. The organism is harbored in the tubular epithelium of the kidneys and is shed in the urine during acute illness and convalescence. Dogs recovered from the "yellows" or Stuttgart's disease have been shown to remain urinary carriers for 4 to 6 months. Through their habits of licking urine and their instinctive interest in each other's genitalia, infection is spread through the nose and tongue directly from dog to dog. Man may acquire the disease through contact with urine of infected dogs or water contaminated with such urine.

In view of the relatively high incidence of infection with *L. canicola* among dogs and their widespread association with man, it is probable that human infection with *L. canicola* is more prevalent than reports tend to indicate. In febrile disease in which the triad of meningeal irritation, conjunctivitis, and albuminuria presents itself, repeated agglutination tests for leptospirosis are therefore indicated.

Note: Attention is called to the fact that serum from the patient examined on November 30, 1952, a period of 2 years after the onset of his illness, still agglutinated with *L. canicola* in a 1:1000 dilution.

REFERENCES

BEAMER, P.R. 1952. Treatment of leptospirosis with antibiotics. Ann. N.Y. Acad. Sci. *55* (art. 6) 1195.

BEESON, P.B. and HANKEY, D.D. 1952. Leptospiral meningitis. AMA Arch. Internal Med. *89*, 575.

BENENSON, A.S. 1975. Control of Communicable Diseases in Man, 12th Edition. American Public Health Association, Washington, D.C.

BIGLER, M.S., COLLINS, T.E., NICHOLS, J.B., GALTON, M.M. and PRATHER, E.C. 1970. Trends of sporadic leptospirosis in Florida. Public Health Rep. *85*, 225.

BROWN, J.C. and MacINTYRE, A.B. 1948. A survey of canine leptospirosis in England. Vet. Rec. *41*, 487.

BRUNNER, T.K. 1949. Canine leptospirosis. North Am. Vet. *30*, 517.

BRYAN, F.L. 1969. Infections due to miscellaneous microorganisms. *In* Foodborne Infections and Intoxications. H. Riemann (Editor). Academic Press, New York.

BUCHANAN, R.E. and GIBBONS, N.E. 1974. Bergey's Manual of Determinative Bacteriology, 8th Edition. Williams & Wilkins Co., Baltimore.

JEGHERS, H. 1953. The leptospiroses in the United States. Bull. N. Engl. Med. Cent. *15*, 61.

14

Other Bacterial Foodborne and Waterborne Diseases

BACILLUS CEREUS FOOD POISONING

Another microorganism found in soil is *Bacillus cereus*, a facultative anaerobic sporeformer that is capable of growing either aerobically or anaerobically and causing gastroenteritis if it is ingested with contaminated vegetables, grains such as rice, and other mishandled foods. Infected persons have intense abdominal colic, vomiting, and diarrhea that lasts for about 24 hr. Outbreaks have been reported in Europe under conditions that permitted multiplication of the bacilli in large numbers.

Diagnosis may be confirmed by the isolation of *B. cereus* from the suspected item of food as well as from the patient's feces, and by culture on special media.

Mild cases with vomiting have an incubation period of 1 to 5 hr; those with diarrhea as the predominant symptom take longer to appear, 6 to 16 hr. As in staphylococcal food poisoning, illness is caused by the action of an enterotoxin produced by the bacillus.

Foods that have had contact with soil, such as vegetables and grains, when cooked, should be kept under proper refrigeration, as spores of *B. cereus* can survive boiling and may multiply rapidly if the cooked food is permitted to remain at room temperature. Leftovers should be reheated in order to avoid multiplication of the organism and the production of its enterotoxin.

Treatment of infected persons is similar to that recommended from staphylococcal food poisoning (see Chapter 4).

VIBRIO PARAHAEMOLYTICUS FOOD POISONING

If 12 to 24 hr after having eaten a seafood dinner, persons develop such symptoms as nausea, vomiting, watery or bloody diarrhea, abdominal cramps, and fever, consideration should be given to the possibility that they have come down with *Vibrio parahaemolyticus* food poisoning.

This is an intestinal disorder caused by *Vibrio parahaemolyticus*, a halophilic spirillum (one that flourishes in a salty environment). Multiple antigenic types of the organism exist with pathogenic strains producing a characteristic hemolytic reaction (a high white blood cell count) known as the "Kamagawa phenomenon." The *Vibrio* is found in marine silt and free in coastal waters and is a natural contaminant of fish and shellfish.

Diagnosis of the illness may be confirmed by blood count and isolation of the virulent strain of the *Vibrio* from the patient's feces. Symptoms occur after the digestion of seafood, raw or cooked insufficiently to destroy the naturally contaminating vibrios. Such food, even when properly cooked, may become cross-contaminated if handled together with raw seafood and if kept improperly refrigerated, permitting sufficient multiplication of the vibrios to cause illness when ingested. It is gratifying that the disease is usually of moderate severity lasting from only 1 to 2 days.

As seafood is the vehicle of transmission of this type of food poisoning, it is important that persons who handle and process it be instructed in its proper cooking, handling, and refrigeration.

Treatment is similar to that for staphylococcal food poisoning—mainly supportive (see Chapter 4).

MELIOIDOSIS

Melioidosis is an uncommon disease that occasionally occurs in parts of Southeast Asia, Australia, and South America. It is caused by *Pseudomonas pseudomalici* also known as Whitmore's bacillus, a saprophytic organism living in soil or water on decaying vegetable matter.

Persons who become infected may be asymptomatic. On the other hand, the disease may prove extremely severe, even fatal. It may simulate tuberculosis, causing pulmonary consolidation, cavitation, chronic lung abscesses, empyema, and osteomyelitis.

It is believed to be transmitted to man by contact with soil or water contaminated with the organism by certain infected animals, such as sheep, goats, swine, horses, and rodents. In humans the bacilli enter the body through an open wound, or by aspiration or ingestion of contaminated water, or by inhalation of dust from soil. The incubation period is uncertain as symptoms may not appear until months or years after exposure.

Diagnosis may be made by the isolation of the causative agent, by agglutination tests, and by fluorescent antibody titers.

Spread may be prevented by the safe disposal of patients' sputum and other discharges, and by the proper care of any overt wound.

The disease responds to treatment with sulfonamides, chloramphenicol, and tetracyclines.

DIPHTHERIA

Brief mention is made of a disease that is rarely seen today, namely, diphtheria, a severe and often fatal disease of the nasopharynx and other mucous membranes.

Although diphtheria is spread primarily by contact with a patient or a carrier, raw milk has served as a vehicle of transmission in the past. However, at present in communities where active immunization of infants and young children with diphtheria toxoid is scrupulously practiced and where milk cannot be sold to the public unless it is processed in accordance with the Standard Grade A Milk Ordinance and is properly pasteurized, diphtheria has been practically eradicated.

Diphtheria has an incubation period of 2 to 5 days. It is caused by *Corynebacterium diphtheriae* that produces a toxin that may cause myocarditis and paralysis of cranial and peripheral motor and sensory nerves. It has a case fatality rate of 5 to 10% and even higher if the laryngeal form occurs in infants and young children, who may succumb to suffocation and to the toxicity.

For those readers who are interested in how a child is protected, the following schedule for primary immunization is given. It should be followed even though no case of diphtheria has occurred in the area for many years.

At 2 or 3 months of age, diphtheria toxoid combined with pertussis (whooping cough) and tetanus toxoid vaccine (DPT) is given in 3 intramuscular injections of 0.5 ml each at intervals of at least 4 weeks and a fourth dose approximately 1 year after the third injection. A booster dose of DPT should be administered when the child is between 3 and 6 years of age and starts to attend school. After 6 years of age, use tetanus and diphtheria toxoids (adult type) (Td). Boosters of Td should be given every 10 years. For the primary immunization of older children not previously immunized, give 2 doses of Td 4 to 6 weeks apart, followed by a reinforcing dose 1 year later.

Patients with diphtheria must be isolated for at least 14 days, or until 2 negative daily nose and throat cultures are obtained after antimicrobial treatment is stopped. All articles soiled by the patient's discharges should be disinfected. Household and other contacts should be quarantined until culture from their noses and throats is free of diphtheria bacilli. Adult contacts whose occupation involves the handling of food or the association with children should be excluded from work until cultures prove that they are no longer carriers.

Siblings of a patient who have been previously immunized should be given a booster dose; if they had no previous immunization, they should receive a primary series of injections. Nose and throat cultures should be taken of contacts in the search for carriers.

If milk is suspected, the dairy and processing plant should be visited and pasteurization records should be inspected for faulty temperatures and timing. Samples should be taken for laboratory examination.

Patients must be treated promptly with diphtheria antitoxin and antibiotics (penicillin and erythromycin). Carriers may be relieved of their condition with the antibiotics (600,000 to 2,000,000 units of aqueous procaine penicillin intramuscularly daily for 10 days, or erythromycin 1.0 g orally for 7 days).

In epidemics, field epidemiologic investigation of reported cases is made in order to identify the source of infection, find contacts, and arrange for the mass immunization of children and other population groups involved.

YERSINIOSIS

In 1973 there occurred in the United States in a rural area with poor sanitary facilities, an outbreak of a severe form of gastroenteritis involving 16 cases, including 2 deaths. The disease was diagnosed as yersiniosis, a form of infection of the intestines and colon caused by *Yersinia enterocolitica* or *Y. pseudotuberculosis*. Infection with the latter organism is considered more lethal, particularly if it occurs in adolescents or the elderly. It is believed to be transmitted from person to person by direct contact, by the fecal-oral route, and by the ingestion of raw foods or water contaminated with animal feces. The incubation period is from 3 to 7 days.

The symptoms of yersiniosis consist of a low-grade fever, anorexia, vomiting, and diarrhea due to an enterocolitis. In addition, patients develop an acute lymphadenitis (enlargement of abdominal lymph nodes) that may be mistaken for acute appendicitis. They may also complain of a pharyngitis, headache, arthritic involvements, the formation of skin nodules, ulcerations, and abscesses, and may come down with septicemia.

The disease occurs in Western Europe, Asia, and Africa with occasional cases or outbreaks reported in the United States. *Y. enterocolitica* has been isolated from the feces of avian and mammalian hosts and recently from primates imported from Africa and the New World. Household pets (cats and dogs) have also been incriminated.

Diagnosis is made by serologic agglutination tests and by the recovery of the infective organism from the feces and from excised tissues.

Prevention of yersiniosis is similar to that for the other diseases spread by the fecal-oral route: sanitary disposal of human and animal (mainly

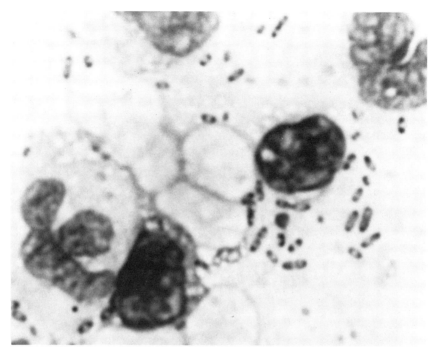

Courtesy of Dr. Hyman Wolochow, Naval Biosciences Laboratory, University of California

FIG. 14.1. IMPRESSION OF SPLEEN FROM A GUINEA PIG INFECTED WITH *YERSINIA PESTIS* (WYSON'S STAIN)

dog) feces, the purification and protection of the water supply from contamination, the sanitary preparation of foods, personal hygiene, handwashing, and the prevention of infected persons from the handling of food.

Although *Yersinia* may be occasionally resistant to penicillin, the other antibiotics such as ampicillin, streptomycin, tetracycline, and chloramphenicol are effective therapeutically.

In discussing the symptoms of *Yersinia*, mention was made that it often closely simulates appendicitis. This was confirmed in an outbreak caused by *Yersinia enterocolitica* that occurred in September 1976, among 218 school children in Oneida County, N.Y., in which chocolate milk was incriminated. A total of 33 of the children were hospitalized for suspected appendicitis, 13 of whom had appendectomies. In each case, at surgery, the appendix was found to be visually and microscopically normal or only slightly inflamed, but mesenteric adenopathy and inflammation of the terminal ilium was observed.

REFERENCES

ASAKAWA, Y. *et al.* 1973. Two community outbreaks of human infection with *Yersinia enterocolitica*. J. Hyg. (Cambridge) *71*, 517.

BARKER, W.H. 1974. *Vibrio parahaemolyticus* outbreaks in the United States. Lancet *1*, 551.

BENENSON, A.S. 1975. Control of Communicable Diseases in Man, 12th Edition. American Public Health Association, Washington, D.C.

BLACK, R.E. *et al.* 1978. Epidemic *Yersinia enterocolitica* infection due to contaminated chocolate milk. N. Engl. J. Med. *298*, 76.

CARRUTHERS, M.M. 1975. Cytotoxicity of *Vibrio parahaemolyticus* in the HeLa cell culture. J. Infect. Dis. *132*, 555.

CRAUN, C.F. and McCABE, L.J. 1973. Review of the causes of waterborne disease outbreaks. J. Am. Water Assoc. *65*, 74.

GOEPFERT, J.M., SPIRA, W.M. and KIM, H.U. 1972. *Bacillus cereus* food poisoning organism. A review. J. Milk Food Technol. *35*, 213.

KOURANY, M. and VASQUEZ, M.A. 1975. The first reported case from Panama of acute gastroenteritis caused by *Vibrio parahaemolyticus*. Am. J. Trop. Med. *24*, 638.

MAXEY, K.E. and ROSENAU, M.J. 1965. Preventive Medicine and Public Health, 9th Edition. P.E. Sartwell (Editor). Appleton-Century-Crofts, New York.

PAI, C.H. and MORS, V. 1978. Production of enterotoxin by *Yersinia enterocolitica*. Infect. Immun. *19*, 908.

PORTNOY, B.L., GOEPFERT, J.M. and HARMON, S.M. 1976. An outbreak of *Bacillus cereus* food poisoning resulting from contaminated vegetable sprouts. Am. J. Epidemiol. *103*, 589.

SMITH, M.R. 1971. *Vibrio parahaemolyticus*. Clin. Med. *78*, 22.

SPECK, M.L. 1976. Compendium of Methods for the Microbiological Examination of Foods. American Public Health Association, Washington, D.C.

TERRANOVA, W. and BLAKE, P.A. 1978. *Bacillus cereus* food poisoning. N. Engl. J. Med. *298*, 143.

TURNBULL, P.C.B. 1976. Studies in the production of enterotoxin by *Bacillus cereus*. J. Clin. Pathol. *29*, 941.

15

Infectious Hepatitis

The term hepatitis refers to inflammation of the liver. There are numerous causes of hepatitis: among them are toxic materials, cirrhosis of the liver, carcinoma of the liver, obstruction of the bile ducts by a calculus (gallstone) or a neoplasm, and the infectious form due to invasion by a virus.

Sources of Infection

The viral form of hepatitis may be caused by 1 of 2 viruses: (1) Virus A that produces a form of hepatitis known as infectious hepatitis, the virus being present in the feces and blood of infected persons, and transmitted orally or parenterally (by needle and syringe), and (2) Virus B, the cause of serum hepatitis that is transmitted only parenterally.

Our attention will be directed solely to the epidemiological and clinical characteristics of infectious hepatitis, caused by Virus A, the form of hepatitis that is foodborne and waterborne.

Infectious hepatitis is not a new disease. It was known in the past as epidemic jaundice and is mentioned in the writings of the Greek physicians of the Hippocratic School, dating it to the 2nd century B.C. Between 1629 and 1868, there were 53 European and 11 American cities that experienced epidemics of hepatitis. During World War II, the disease reached tremendous proportions with more than 170,000 cases recorded in the United States Army. The cause of these epidemics was unknown until it was demonstrated several decades ago that a virus was responsible for the disease.

Infectious hepatitis is spread by person-to-person contact through the fecal-oral route by an infected person harboring Virus A in his feces or urine. Epidemics result, as they do with the bacterial foodborne and waterborne diseases, because of common exposure to contaminated food, milk, water, or raw shellfish from polluted waters.

Characteristics

Hepatitis A virus is excreted in the feces of infected persons during the second half of the incubation period and during the preicteric phase (before jaundice sets in). It persists for 1 to 2 weeks after the appearance of jaundice.

The onset of illness is abrupt, with fever, headache, lassitude, malaise, anorexia, nausea, vomiting, and abdominal discomfort with tenderness over the liver. It is soon followed by jaundice, brownish urine, and clay colored feces. In adults the severity of illness increases with age. It may be mild and last from 1 to 2 weeks, or it may become severely disabling and last for several months. During convalescence, patients remain easily fatigued and complain of lassitude and loss of appetite. The disease is usually milder in children and is often anicteric (without jaundice).

Its incubation period is rather prolonged, from 10 to 50 days, commonly 30 to 35 days. It is seen more frequently in rural areas than in cities and occurs usually in the spring and summer. Outbreaks have been reported in institutions, military camps, and low-cost housing projects. Its case fatality rate during epidemics is exceedingly low.

Prevention and Control

As infectious hepatitis, like the other foodborne and waterborne diseases, spreads through the fecal-oral route, it may be prevented by proper sanitation and personal hygiene with emphasis on the proper disposal of feces and urine and on the purification and protection of the water supply. One should refrain from eating raw shellfish (oysters and clams) that have been gathered from questionable sources as their infection with hepatitis virus-bearing sewage is a probability. Travelers to endemic areas, such as the Middle East and Africa, should receive passive immunization with immune gamma globulin (0.02 ml per kg of body weight) for a short exposure, or 3 times the dose for a prolonged stay with repeated injections every 4 to 6 months). With the virus being also present in the blood, any needle or syringe used on patients must be thoroughly sterilized by autoclaving for 30 min at 121.5°C (15 psi or 103.5 Pa pressure), or by dry heat for 2 hr, or by boiling in water for 30 min.

Cases of infectious hepatitis must be reported to the health department. Spread of the disease may be prevented by: (1) isolating patients during the first 2 weeks of illness and for 1 week after the onset of jaundice; (2) restricting sick food handlers as is done in the other foodborne diseases; (3) disposing of patient's feces and urine in a sanitary manner; and (4) inoculating contacts with immune gamma globulin intramuscularly (0.02 ml per kg of body weight) as soon as possible after exposure. The gamma globulin is prepared from pools of human plasma derived from 10,000 to 25,000 blood donors.

Epidemiologic investigation should be made of all outbreaks in order to find a common source of infection and to determine the mode of transmission. A search should be made for illness among suspected food handlers. Corrective steps must be taken to prevent further contamination of the food or water found to have been responsible for the outbreak. Institutional outbreaks will require mass prophylactic immunization of contacts with immune gamma globulin.

Diagnosis

The diagnosis of infectious hepatitis may be confirmed by the following liver function tests performed by the laboratory:

(1) Serum bilirubin determination to diagnose icteric illness and its severity.
(2) Icteric index to follow the course of jaundice.
(3) Cephalin flocculation to quantitatively determine alterations in serum protein due to liver disease.
(4) Thymal turbidity that indicates what injury the liver has sustained.
(5) Urine bilirubin and urobilinogen determination indicating injury to the kidneys.
(6) Serum transaminase: glutamic-oxalacetic transminase (SGOT) helps in making a differential diagnosis of viral hepatitis (SGOT level in healthy persons is 40 to 110 units; in infected persons it may go to 1000 to 2000 units during the acute phase).

Treatment

Treatment for infectious hepatitis is symptomatic and nonspecific. The patient needs complete bed rest. His diet should be simple and palatable, of adequate caloric intake, and high in protein and dairy fats. It may be necessary to administer 10% glucose solution intravenously to supplement oral intake. Antihistamines may be given for the relief of nausea. During convalescence, the patient should be served a full, unrestricted, well-balanced diet containing from 3000 to 4000 calories.

A description of a foodborne outbreak of infectious hepatitis that occurred in Nassau County and was investigated by the authors follows. It should prove instructive as it illustrates how the information given in the text may be put to practical use.

OUTBREAK OF INFECTIOUS HEPATITIS

Previous to November 1, 1965, few cases of infectious hepatitis had been reported in the villages of Elmont and Valley Stream in Nassau County, N.Y., but since January 1, 1965, physicians had reported a total of 5 such cases in Elmont and 11 cases in Valley Stream. During the whole of 1964 only 3 cases had been reported in Elmont and 9 in Valley Stream, a respective annual rate of 9.7 and 14.2 per 100,000 population for the 2 villages.

Early in November, however, numerous reports began to come in from physicians and hospitals serving Elmont and a portion of Valley Stream known as North Valley Stream. The areas in question have a combined population of 22,100 persons. Subsequently, a total of 90 such reports was received, 65 from Elmont and 25 from North Valley Stream, resulting in a combined rate of 407.2 cases per 100,000 population. These included 10 persons who, although residing in other parts of the county, appear to have become infected in Elmont.

When studied by dates of onset of illness, the reports revealed that the outbreak began the week of September 12. There was a sharply rising and falling curve with 74 cases occurring between the middle of October and the middle of November over a period of approximately 5 weeks.

The predominance of cases, 48 in number, occurred in young persons 19 years and under (the youngest being 7 years old); and 42 cases were among adults, 20 of them being over 40 years of age. The sex distribution was 58.9% males and 41.1% females.

When the addresses of the reported cases were spotted on a street map of Elmont and Valley Stream, it was found that they were clustered immediately north and south of Dutch Broadway, a main thoroughfare in Elmont, over a distance of about 3.2 km (2 mi) (Fig. 15.1). In order to determine whether a similar increase in incidence of hepatitis had occurred in Queens County, the New York City Department of Health was contacted. They reported that there was no significant increase of such cases in the area of Queens adjacent to Elmont.

The clustering of cases over a short period of time in a limited area strongly suggested a common-source exposure. As common-source outbreaks of infectious hepatitis have been known to be waterborne, milkborne, or foodborne, these possibilities were given consideration.

Water Supply

The area in question receives its water from Jamaica Water Supply Company which supplies approximately 530,000 residents in Queens County and 130,000 persons in Nassau County residing in Elmont, North Valley Stream, Floral Park, Bellerose, New Hyde Park, and a portion

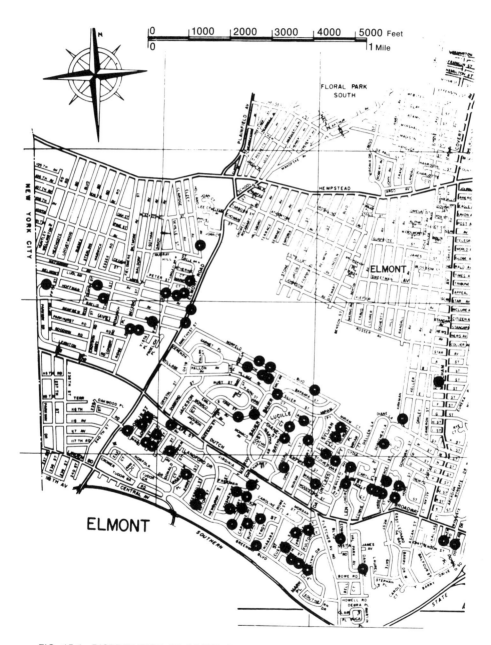

FIG. 15.1. DISTRIBUTION OF CASES OF
INFECTIOUS HEPATITIS IN ELMONT, N.Y., 1965

of Garden City. The entire system is one integrated network with well fields and storage fairly uniformly distributed throughout the franchised area. The water supply is totally from wells, 23 of which are located in Nassau County with depths ranging from 26 m (85 ft) to 221.5 m (727 ft). Routine chlorination with a dose of approximately 0.1 ppm is practiced at every well. The Dutch Broadway area is served by water from any of 5 stations or well fields, depending on system demand. Well Field 28, which is located roughly in the center of the area, contains 2 wells, 27 m (89 ft) and 157 m (514 ft) in depth, and a 5.7 million liter (1.5 million gal.) elevated storage tank.

Treatment at the site consists of lime addition and chlorination. Bacteriologic samples taken on November 10, including 1 sample from the water tank and 10 distribution system samples from various points in and about the region in question, proved satisfactory.

A check of Health Department records indicated that no sample positive for coliforms had been obtained from the Jamaica Water Supply Company's distribution system since June 1965. With the exception of minor service leaks, no main break had occurred previous to August. These findings, plus the wide distribution of the system both in Nassau and Queens counties, tended to rule out the water supply as a possible source of transmission.

Questionnaire

A detailed questionnaire was prepared with the intention of visiting each patient and securing pertinent epidemiologic information. It was possible to interview and complete questionnaires on all but 3 patients. Analysis of the information revealed the following:

(1) Signs and symptoms of practically each patient were consistent with the diagnosis of infectious hepatitis; laboratory examinations confirmed existing impairment of liver function.
(2) There were 7 anicteric cases, all but 1 in children.
(3) 41 patients were admitted to hospitals.
(4) Raw shellfish has been eaten by only 15 patients at different establishments within 2 months prior to onset of illness.
(5) No gathering, party, dinner, or banquet was attended in common by the patients.
(6) No supermarket where food was purchased was named in common or in significant frequency by the patients.
(7) 23 patients stated that they had received some type of parenteral injection, and 8 had novocaine injections preparatory to dental extractions by various physicians and dentists during the time consistent with the incubation period of the disease. This would

tend to rule out the possibility of so-called "syringe hepatitis" outbreak.

(8) Patients named 20 dairies or food markets as the source of their
milk supply. However, 42 patients (48.5%) stated that they obtained their milk from Gouz Dairy.

(9) When the patients were questioned as to where they had purchased
cold cuts, sliced meats, or salads within the past 2 months, they
named 9 various delicatessens and groceries.

Of the 76 cases with dates of onset between October 13 and November
21, 66 (86.8%) had purchased these foods from Delicatessen Store A in
the preceding 2 months. Six patients (7.0%) named Delicatessen Store B.

The 2 findings which appeared to require further investigation were
Gouz Dairy and Delicatessen Store A.

Gouz Dairy

This dairy is a milk pasteurization and bottling plant located on Dutch
Broadway. It has a self-service store where customers pick up 0.95 liter
(1 qt) bottles of whole milk, skimmed milk, buttermilk, chocolate milk,
orange juice, apple cider, punch drinks, and eggs, pay the cashier, and
carry the purchases to their cars. As these products are sold at reduced
prices (19¢ per 0.95 liter or 1 qt of milk), the dairy is patronized by a
great number of residents of that area. The management stated that
from 28,000 to 40,000 quarts of milk are sold daily, the bulk of it, about
80%, to persons residing in Queens. Milk, milk products, and orange juice
are pasteurized on the premises.

Inspection of the pasteurization and storage equipment by our chief
sanitarian revealed it to be in good sanitary and operating condition.
On reviewing the dairy's pasteurization temperature recording charts for
the past 3 months, no evidence of any failure in pasteurization technique
was found. Milk is pasteurized by the H.T.S.T. (High Temperature Short
Time) method at 71°C (160°F) or over and cooled to 3.9° or 4.4°C (39°
or 40°F).

The bottle washing and filling operation and the storage of bottled
milk were also found to be satisfactory. According to the management,
no serious or prolonged illness had occurred among the employees of the
dairy during the past 3 months.

Although nearly half of the patients with hepatitis had patronized this
dairy because of its proximity to their home and the cut-rate prices,
no evidence could be found to incriminate it. Besides, there had been
no increase in the incidence of cases of hepatitis in Queens where the
major part of the dairy's milk is consumed.

Delicatessen Store A

This establishment was located on Dutch Broadway, a short distance from Gouz Dairy and was owned by R.S., who resided in Jamaica, Queens. He had been an employee of the store during 1964 and had acquired ownership to it on April 1, 1965. He employed 2 clerks to assist him. Cooked meats and meat products sold at the store were purchased from known and reliable wholesalers. R.S. personally prepared the various salads, sliced the cold cuts, and served customers from behind the counter. Among the items prepared and sold were rice pudding, potato salad, macaroni salad, cole slaw, health salad (a mixture of fresh vegetables), baked custard, meat cakes, Virginia ham, roast beef, fish cakes, and clam chowder. The clams used in the chowder were either canned or purchased from a local supermarket.

On questioning the persons operating the store, it was learned that the clerks had been in good health for the past 6 months. The owner, however, stated that on about October 1st he had an illness characterized by fever, malaise, headache, tenderness over the region of the liver, clay-colored stools, and jaundice. Although he could not give a definite date of onset of illness, he stated that he had not felt entirely well for several weeks prior to October 1st. His family physician, whom he visited on October 13, made some liver function tests and found an elevated bilirubin—total 7.5 mg %, indirect 4.45 mg %, a positive urobilinogen, and an increased serum transaminase (SGPT 402.0 units). The physician diagnosed the illness as billiary obstruction due to gallstones. R.S. continued to work in the store until October 16, preparing various salads, slicing meats, and serving customers. At his physician's instructions, he remained at home for a period of 18 days, although he visited the store periodically during that time, allegedly for purposes of bookkeeping. He returned to work and resumed his duties on November 3.

Delicatessen Store B

This store, located about 1.2 km (0.75 mi) from Delicatessen Store A, was owned and operated by P.E., who shared an apartment with R.S. When interviewed on November 23, he appeared in good health and denied any recent illness. R.S. stated that he had given P.E. financial assistance in acquiring the store and that on September 8 and September 9 he had assisted P.E. by waiting on customers between the hours of 6 and 9 P.M.

Control Group

In order to determine to what extent residents of that area normally patronized Delicatessen Store A, and whether there was significance to the finding that 88.6% of the persons who developed hepatitis had eaten food products purchased from that store, a sample of 94 persons residing in that area who had not been reported as having hepatitis were questioned as to where they purchased salads and cold cuts. The homes selected were located on the same streets as those of persons with hepatitis. It was found that only 15 of them, or 17.0%, had patronized Delicatessen Store A within the past 3 months.

When persons in the control group were questioned as to the source of their milk supply, 37.2% stated that they regularly purchased milk from Gouz Dairy. Among the patients with hepatitis, 48.5% obtained their milk from the same dairy. Perhaps this discrepancy is due to the fact that the dairy is located a few stores away from Delicatessen Store A and consequently customers of one would find it convenient to patronize the other.

Discussion and Conclusions

With the occurrence of a large proportion of cases in a limited geographic area within a short period of time, the outbreak may be considered to be due to a common source of infection. Interview with the patients indicated that the outbreak was most probably foodborne and that the majority had eaten food purchased from one source, namely, Delicatessen Store A.

It is our opinion, after discussing R.S.'s illness with his physician, that he had suffered a moderately severe attack of infectious hepatitis rather than chololithiasis; and that he most probably contaminated one or more of the foods he prepared and handled in the store during the infectious period of his illness, thus spreading hepatitis virus among his customers and infecting those who were susceptible to the disease. On questioning, he could not pinpoint the exact day he first began to feel sick. He hinted that late in July he had had an "upset stomach" with several recurrent periods of abdominal pain. The pain became worse on about October 1, at which time he developed characteristic symptoms of infectious hepatitis.

The incubation period of infectious hepatitis is given as from 15 to 50 days, with an average of about 25 days. Human volunteer studies indicate that the virus appears in the feces during the preicteric phase of the illness and persists for 1 to 2 weeks after the onset of jaundice in the typical adult case. The virus is also excreted in the stools late in the incubation period.

The 6 persons who also ate food purchased from Delicatessen Store B became ill from 6 to 8 weeks after September 8 and 9, on which days R.S. admitted assisting in that store. If he were the one responsible for their illness, it would appear that he was also infectious at that time. He could have been shedding hepatitis virus while preparing salads and slicing meats in his own store from that date until after the appearance of jaundice on October 13.

Additional confirmatory evidence pointing to R.S. as the most probable source of infection was found in 10 persons who reside in other villages in the county some distance from Delicatessen Stores A and B. They had either purchased and eaten salads or cold cuts from those stores or had partaken of similarly obtained foods in the homes of Elmont residents.

If the patients who purchased food from both delicatessen stores are added together, then it is found that R.S. appears responsible for an attack rate of 88.5%. Of the remaining 11.5% who did not eat food from either store, 9 of them (10.5%) indicated that they had had contact with one or more of the foodborne cases outside their own household. They may be considered secondary cases; none of them, however, resided in the same household as the reported cases, and none had received immune gamma globulin prophylactically.

Control Measures

Gamma globulin was issued by this department for the protection of household contacts of infected cases. A total of 642 ml of globulin was distributed to physicians for the injection of 393 such contacts in 58 households. It was anticipated that this would minimize to a considerable degree the number of secondary cases which usually follow hepatitis outbreaks as shown in previous studies. Our hopes were realized as no secondary case occurred in any of the households.

On November 13, when evidence began to suggest that R.S. might be the source of infection of the reported cases, he was instructed to stay away from the store until further notice. The sanitary inspector assigned to that area was instructed to make daily visits at irregular times to ascertain that he complied with that order.

In view of the lack of definite knowledge as to how long a convalescing patient continues to excrete the virus in his feces after recovery and the absence of a specific laboratory test helpful in making such a determination, the question arose as to how long R.S. should be prohibited from engaging in his occupation. As a food handler, his premature return to work could continue to endanger the community. On the other hand, it would appear unjust to prevent him from earning his livelihood over an unnecessarily prolonged period of time because we did not know the exact length of the period of infectivity of this disease.

Although the Department of Health had at no time released the information to the public as to which store or what person was responsible for the outbreak, it was common knowledge among R.S.'s customers that he had been ill. His jaundiced condition had been noticed by some, and a rumor had spread that he had hepatitis and had caused the illness among his customers. Consequently, business at the store dropped to a standstill. In view of this, and the anticipation of future financial losses, R.S. decided to return his store to its former owner and to go into bankruptcy. He was uncertain as to his plans for the future.

On negotiating with his creditor, no satisfactory agreement was reached. However, when the creditor offered certain substantial financial inducements if R.S. would continue to operate the store, he decided to accept the offer.

It is gratifying to report that the last case reported in the Elmont and North Valley Stream area had an onset on November 21, and no additional case incriminating either Delicatessen Store A or B has been reported since that date.

REFERENCES

ASHLEY, A. 1954. Gamma globulin. Effect on secondary attack rates of infectious hepatitis. N. Engl. J. Med. *250*, 412.

BATIK, O., CRAUN, G.F., TUTHILL, R.W. and KRAEME, D.F. 1980. An epidemiologic study of the relationship between hepatitis A and water supply characteristics and treatment. Am. J. Public Health *70*, 167.

BROOKS, B.D., HSIA, D.Y.Y. and GELLIS, S.S. 1953. Family outbreaks of infectious hepatitis: Prophylactic use of gamma globulin. N. Engl. J. Med. *249*, 58.

CLARK, W., SACKS, D. and WILLIAMS, H. 1955. An outbreak of infectious hepatitis on a college campus. Am. J. Trop. Med. *7*, 263.

CLARKE, N.A. et al. 1975. Virus study for drinking water supplies. J. Am. Water Works Assoc. *67*, 192.

CLIVER, D.O. 1971. Transmission of viruses through foods. Crit. Rev. Environ. Control. *1* (4) 551.

CRAUN, G.E. and McCABE, L.J. 1973. Review of the causes of waterborne disease outbreaks. J. Am. Water Works Assoc. *65*, 74.

DENES, A.E. et al. 1977. Foodborne hepatitis A infection. A report of two urban restaurant-associated outbreaks. Am. J. Epidemiol. *105*, 156.

DOUGHERTY, W.J. and ALTMAN, R. 1962. Viral hepatitis in New Jersey, 1960–1961. Am. J. Med. *32*, 104.

DULL, H.B., DOEGE, T.C. and MOSLEY, J.W. 1963. An outbreak of infectious hepatitis associated with a school cafeteria. South. Med. J. *56*, 475.

HERMANN, J.E., KOSTONBADER, K.D., JR. and CLIVER, C.O. 1974. Persistance of enteroviruses in lake water. Appl. Microbiol. *28*, 895.

HUGHES, J.M., MORSON, M.H. and GANGAROSA, E.J. 1977. The safety of eating shellfish. J. Am. Med. Assoc. *237*, 1980.

JOSEPH, P.R., MILLER, J.D. and HENDERSON, D.A. 1965. An outbreak of hepatitis traced to food contamination. N. Engl. J. Med. *273*, 188.

KRUGMAN, S., WARD, R. and GILES, J.P. 1962. The natural history of infectious hepatitis. Am. J. Med *32*, 717.

LEGER, R.T. *et al.* 1975. Hepatitis A. Report of a common source oubreak with recovery of a possible etiologic agent. I. Epidemiologic studies. J. Infect. Dis. *131*, 163.

MASON, J.D. and McLEAN, W.R. 1962. Infectious hepatitis traced to the consumption of raw oysters. Am. J. Hyg. *75*, 90.

McCOLLUM, R.W. 1961. An outbreak of viral hepatitis in the Mediterranean Fleet. Mil. Med. *126*, 902.

McCOLLUM, R.W. 1962. Epidemiologic patterns of viral hepatitis. Am. J. Med. *32*, , 657.

MOSLEY, J.W. 1971. Viral hepatitis: A group of epidemiologic entities. Can. Med. Assoc. J. *106*, 427.

NOBLE, H.B. and PETERSON, D.R. 1965. Evaluation of immune serum globulin for control of infectious hepatitis. Public Health Rep. *80*, 173.

STOKES, J., JR. 1960. Viral Hepatitis. Pediatr. Clin. North Am. 7 (4) 989.

STOKES, J., JR. 1962. The control of viral hepatitis. Am. J. Med. *32*, 729.

STOKES, J., JR. *et al.* 1954. The carrier state in viral hepatitis. J. Am. Med. Assoc. *154*, 1059.

SUMMERSKILL, W.H.J. 1962. Anicteric hepatitis. J. Am. Med. Assoc. *182*, 1336.

TARTAKOW, I.J. 1977. Casebook of a medical detective: A review of interesting cases. Nassau County Med. Cent. *4* (2) 65–73.

TAYLOR, F.B. *et al.* 1966. The case for waterborne hepatitis. Am. J. Public Health *56*, 2093.

WARD, R., KRUGMAN, S. and GILES, J.P. 1960. Etiology and prevention of infectious hepatitis. Postgrad. Med. *28*, 12.

16

Other Viral Foodborne and Waterborne Diseases

The report to the surgeon general in 1962 of the Commission on Environmental Health Problems that consisted of public health experts contains the following statement:

> More than 70 viruses have been detected in human feces. All may be present in sewage. Viruses pass through sewage treatment plants, persist in contaminated waters, and may penetrate the water treatment plants. Numerous outbreaks of infectious hepatitis have been traced to contaminated drinking water. The occurence of such incidents appears to be increasing.

As to other alleged waterborne viral diseases, there is inconclusive evidence to include any viral disease other than infectious hepatitis in that category. On noting the number of published reports of waterborne outbreaks of poliomelitis, Mosley (1965) made a scholarly analysis of 8 such reports. He concluded that with only one possible exception, sufficient data to suggest that waterborne transmission of poliomyelitis was responsible for the outbreaks were lacking. The exception is the report by Bancroft *et al.* (1957) of an outbreak that occurred in 1952 in Huskerville, Nebraska.

There are, however, several viral diseases that are believed to be foodborne. Two such diseases, lymphocytic choriomeningitis and hemorrhagic fever, will be discussed. Rodents serve as the reservoir of infection for humans in both instances. A third disease is a form of viral gastroenteritis spread by contaminated human feces.

LYMPHOCYTIC CHORIOMENINGITIS

Urine and feces of mice may contain a virus that causes lymphocytic choriomeningitis if the aforementioned excreta contaminate food eaten by man. Illness may start with an influenza-like attack in 8 to 13 days after the contaminated food is ingested. The patient either recovers completely, or 15 to 21 days after onset, signs of meningoencephalitis of the disease, ranging from 5 to 30% and being greatest among older males.

Laboratory diagnosis is made by the isolation of the virus from the blood or throat washings, and serologically by complement fixation or neutralization tests.

Once the disease occurs, further spread may be prevented by specific rodent control where the reservoir host has been identified.

VIRAL GASTROENTERITIS

There are 2 known types of viral gastroenteritis in which man serves as the reservoir of infection: (1) the milder epidemic type that is believed to be caused by a parvovirus (27 nm particle) occurs mostly in outbreaks among adults during the winter months, and (2) the more severe sporadic form associated with a reovirus-like (70 nm) particle is seen primarily in infants and young children. Both etiologic viruses may be identified from fecal preparations from patients by immune electron microscopy and by serologic tests.

Epidemic viral gastroenteritis is characterized by fever, malaise, nausea, vomiting, abdominal pain, and diarrhea. It has an incubation period of 1 to 2 days. Illness is self-limited, lasting from 24 to 48 hr. One attack is believed to confer immunity to the same viral serotype.

The sporadic type of viral gastroenteritis that attacks the very young occurs sporadically or in outbreaks. It has an incubation period of less than 48 hr, and sick infants develop fever and diarrhea with occasional vomiting.

As viral gastroenteritis is believed to be spread by the fecal-oral route, hygienic measures that are applicable to that type of transmission are recommended. It is also important to avoid exposure of infants and young children to persons with gastrointestinal symptoms.

REFERENCES

BANCROFT, P.M., ENGLEHARD, W.E. and EVANS, C.A. 1957. Poliomyelitis in Huskerville (Lincoln) Nebraska. J. Am. Med. Assoc. *164*, 836.

BENENSON, A.S. 1975. Control of Communicable Diseases in Man, 12th Edition. American Public Health Association, Washington, D.C.

CLARK, N.A. *et al.* 1975. Virus study for drinking water supplies. J. Am. Water Works Assoc. *67*, 192.

CLIVER, D.O. 1971. Transmission of viruses through food. Crit. Rev. Environ. Control *1*, 551.

KOSTENBADER, K.D. and CLIVER, D.O. 1977. Quest for viruses associated with food supply. J. Food Sci. *42*, 1253.

(inflammation of the brain and its membranes) may appear with somnolence (drowsiness), disturbed deep reflexes, paralysis, and anesthesia of the skin. Recovery usually occurs within several weeks, although severe cases occasionally prove fatal. Diagnosis may be confirmed by (1) examination of the spinal fluid that may contain from several hundred to 3500 cells (mostly lymphocytes) per mm^3; (2) isolation of the virus from the patient's blood, urine, nasopharynx, or spinal fluid by inoculation into guinea pigs or mice; (3) occurrence of a rising titer of neutralizing or complement-fixation antibodies in paired sera.

Although the disease is uncommon, foci of infection have been found to persist within the limits of a city block for months or years, causing sporadic cases. The infected house mouse, *Mus musculus*, serves as the main reservoir of infection. It carries the virus for life and excretes it in its urine and feces. The female mouse transmits the virus to its offspring, thus perpetuating the disease. Monkeys, dogs, swine, and guinea pigs have also been incriminated.

It is obvious that the disease may be prevented by cleanliness of the home and place of employment, by the elimination of mice within the home, and by the disposal of other diseased animals.

Spread may be prevented when caring for a person with lymphocytic choriomeningitis by proper disposal of his urine and feces, and by the disinfection of discharges from his nose and throat and of articles soiled therewith.

HEMORRHAGIC FEVER

During the autumn and winter of 1955, laborers working in the cornfields in Argentina came down with a fever that was associated with severe hemorrhagic symptoms. Subsequently, similar epidemics were reported in several small villages in Bolivia. Epidemiologic investigations incriminated wild rodents in the cornfields as the reservoir of infection in Argentina, and domestic rodents in Bolivia.

The incubation period of hemorrhagic fever is from 10 to 14 days. Its onset is gradual, with fever and sweats, malaise and headache, followed by prostration with decreased heart rate, lowered blood pressure, and reduced leucocyte count. Several days after onset, a skin eruption appears on the thorax and flanks. The hemorrhagic manifestations of the disease that occur as it increases in severity consist of petechiae (hemorrhagic spots) in the skin and mucous membranes of the mouth, followed by gingival hemorrhage (bleeding of the gums), epistaxis (nosebleed), melena (dark colored, tarry stools due to the presence of blood altered by the intestinal juices), and hematuria (passage of blood in the urine). Illness lasts from 1 to 2 weeks and its case fatality rate depends on the severity

MOSLEY, J.W. 1965. Transmission of viral diseases by drinking water. *In* Transmission of Viruses by the Water Route. G. Berg (Editor). John Wiley & Sons, New York.

U.S. DEP. HEALTH, EDUC. WELFARE. 1962. Report of the Commission on Environmental Health Problems to the Surgeon General. U.S. Public Health Service Publ. *908*. U.S. Govt. Printing Office, Washington, D.C.

WILNER, B.I. 1969. Classification of the Major Groups of Human and Other Animal Viruses, 4th Edition. Burgess, Minneapolis.

17

Protozoan Intestinal Infections

AMEBIASIS

Sabbatical leave is defined in *Webster's Dictionary* as a "leave of absence granted every seventh year, as to a college professor, for rest, travel, or research." This is based on the practice that was observed many years ago in Ancient Judea of permitting cultivated land to remain idle during the growing season every seventh year in order to permit it to regenerate and prove more productive for the following 7 years. Educators, apparently, feel that the human brain should similarly be allowed to fallow for the same reason.

D.C., an art teacher at a high school in Nassau County, was determined to achieve all 3 aims during his sabbatical leave: he would rest from his daily classroom routine, and travel to the Orient where he would do research in ancient architecture which he greatly admired. Japan, Indonesia, Singapore, and India were the countries he planned to visit.

Although his leave proved inspiring and instructive, he paid dearly for it as far as his own health and that of his wife, who accompanied him, were concerned. While in Japan visiting several Shinto shrines located in rural areas where malaria was endemic, D.C. came down with the disease for which he received antimalarial medication with favorable result. Two months later in India, he and his wife had several attacks of bloody diarrhea while visiting an ancient temple in a remote area. Their illness was diagnosed as an infestation of intestinal parasites. They received anti-helminthic drugs and expelled large quantities of worms by rectum. As the diarrhea persisted, further examination revealed that they both also had acquired amebiasis. On their return home, upon microscopic examination of their feces, *Entamoeba histolytica* was isolated. Treatment with emetine hydrochloride and tetracycline was administered to them.

Had Mr. and Mrs. D.C. consulted the department of health previous to their trip, they might have been spared their unfortunate experience and

127

would have enjoyed their architectural pilgrimage more. Prophylactic treatment for amebiasis and suppression of malaria would have been recommended to them. Starting 2 weeks before their trip, they would have been advised to take a weekly oral dose of 3 tablets of Millibus with Aralen (Winthrop) daily for 2 successive days and continue the same course of treatment during their stay in any infested area where sanitary conditions are poor. Millibus is a brand of glycobiarsol and is amebicidal, and Aralen is a brand of chloroquin which is a malarial suppressant.

Amebiasis, once considered to be a disease of the tropics, is now seen in populations throughout the world. It occurs in persons living under poor hygienic conditions, in institutions, mental hospitals, orphanages, prisons, and in troops in combat. Although in the United States its highest incidence is in rural areas of the southern states among the lower socioeconomic groups, it may also occur among any groups of people. This was demonstrated in 1933 when a major epidemic of amebiasis occurred in Chicago due to defective plumbing that permitted contamination of the drinking water supply with sewage of a large hotel.

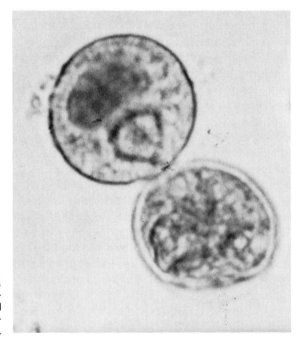

FIG. 17.1. *ENTAMOEBA HISTOLYTICA*. IODINE-STAINED CYST FROM ZINC SULFATE CONCENTRATE OF STOOL

Courtesy of Elliot Scientific Corp. and Abbott Laboratories

Amebiasis or amebic dysentery is a disease of the large intestine due to the invasion of its mucosa by *Entamoeba histolytica*, a pathogenic protozoan that undergoes the following life cycle:

(1) Mature cysts of the ameba are ingested in food contaminated by a subclinical case or a carrier of amebiasis, or in water polluted by sewage.

(2) The cysts pass intact from the stomach to the small intestine.

(3) Alkaline digestive juices in the small intestine activate the cysts and mobile trophozoites emerge and are carried in the fecal stream to the cecum.

(4) The active trophozoites in the cecum multiply by binary fission and invade the intestinal wall, ulcerating it to the submucosa by cytolytic action.

(5) The trophozoites enter the feces and as they travel along the colon, they secrete a cell wall and become cysts.

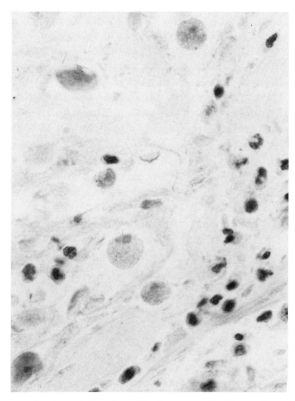

FIG. 17.2. *E. HISTOLYTICA*. INTESTINAL AMEBIASIS: SECTION OF INTESTINAL MUCOSA SHOWING CLUSTERS OF TROPHOZOITES

Courtesy of Elliot Scientific Corp. and Abbott Laboratories

(6) The cysts are excreted in the feces and infect new hosts by contaminating food or water.

(7) As trophozoites are fragile and die rapidly upon exposure to changes in temperature outside the colon, it is the cysts that are responsible for the spread of the disease.

(8) While in the colon, trophozoites may be carried via the portal bloodstream from the intestinal lesions to the liver where they may form an abscess that may perforate into the peritoneal cavity or lung. These complications may occur even in the atypical cases.

The incubation period of amebiasis is from 5 days to several months, commonly 3 to 4 weeks. Symptoms depend upon the degree of infection and the response of the patient. Illness may be asymptomatic or mild with abdominal discomfort, distension, and diarrhea alternating with constipation. In severe cases, diarrhea may be more profuse with blood and mucus, dehydration, and blood loss. Diagnosis is made by fecal examination and the identification of cysts. If the examination is made while the feces are still warm, it is possible to observe the motile trophozoites.

The mild or asymptomatic cases constitute the main source of infection, as often these cases tend to become chronic and continue to shed cysts in the feces for long periods of time. Spread is made by contamination of foods by hands soiled with fresh feces containing trophozoites or spores. Raw vegetables are vulnerable, particularly if night soil (human excreta) is used as fertilizer, an unsanitary practice still in use by some truck farmers. Flies may also spread the disease as cysts have been found in their droppings.

Measures for the prevention of amebiasis are similar to those recommended for other foodborne and waterborne diseases:

(1) Sanitary disposal of feces.

(2) Protection of public water supplies against fecal contamination. Spread may take place when a closed water supply is grossly contaminated with sewage in areas that utilize open brooks and wells that can be readily polluted. As *E. histolytica* cysts are not destroyed by the concentration of chlorination ordinarily used in water treatment, boiling of water may be necessary. Cysts may be removed by use of diatomaceous filters. Cross connections between water supplies and backflow connections in plumbing systems must be avoided.

(3) Health education of the general public, as well as food handlers, in hygiene such as handwashing after defecation and before preparing food.

(4) Inspection and supervision of health and sanitary practices in public eating establishments.
(5) Protection of food from fly contamination.

Cases and epidemics of amebiasis should be reported to the health department so that they may be promptly investigated to determine their source of infection and mode of transmission (food or water). If food is found to be contaminated, its sale should be prohibited or it should be destroyed. If water is suspected, any improper unapproved sanitary plumbing installation, if discovered, should be promptly eliminated.

As it appears that no regimen of treatment for amebiasis is invariably successful, there is controversy as to which of the recommended medications should be used. A number of them are capable of eradicating the amebae in the intestinal lumen, but have little or no effect on extra-intestinal infection such as liver abscess. With other remedies the reverse is true. Consequently, as individually they are not entirely effective, it is necessary to use combinations of medications.

The general treatment for amebiasis is supportive. Rest in bed, control of diet, infusions and transfusions to restore fluid and blood levels are recommended. Broad spectrum antibiotics often have a dramatic symptomatic effect and tend to control the diarrhea by attacking secondary bacterial infection of the intestinal tract. As even asymptomatic cases may have extensive amebic ulcerations in the colon, they should also receive treatment, not only as a public health potential problem but as a benefit to themselves.

The amebicides that are used for intestinal amebiasis with various degrees of success consist of metronidazole (Flagyl), paromomycin (Humatin), tetracycline, or emetine hydrochloride. The latter may relieve symptoms but will not eliminate the infection and should therefore be accompanied or followed by Diodoquin, carbarsone, Milibis, Entero-vioform or emetine bismuth iodide.

For extra-intestinal amebiasis (liver or lung abscess), Flagyl, Aralen, or emetine hydrochloride should be administered. If aspiration of the abscess is to be done, it should be preceded by a course of chloroquin or emetine to limit infection.

In order to ascertain that complete eradication of the amebae in the intestine has been achieved, follow-up fecal examinations should be made every 3 to 6 months until no amebae are found. If a relapse occurs, then the course of treatment should be repeated.

GIARDIASIS

Twenty-three waterborne outbreaks of giardiasis were reported in the United States between 1972 and 1977. During 1979, outbreaks occurred in California, Colorado, Oregon, and Pennsylvania among people who drank contaminated water (U.S. Dep. Health, Educ. Welfare, Cent. Dis. Control 1980).

Giardiasis is an infection of the small intestine caused by *Giardia lamblia*, a flagellated protozoan. Light infections are usually asymptomatic. With heavy infestation, there is damage to the intestinal mucosa causing patients to complain of abdominal cramps, bloating, chronic diarrhea with greasy malodorous stools due to malabsorption of fats, anemia, fatigue, and weight loss. Large numbers of protozoa are excreted in the feces.

The disease is diagnosed by identifying cysts or trophozoites (the vegetative form as distinguished from the reproductive form of the protozoan) in the feces. It is important to look for cysts as the adult forms and the trophozoites are fragile and do not survive outside the body of the host. Children in areas of poor sanitation and in institutions are more frequently infected than adults. In the United States, the carrier rate ranges from 1.5 to 20%.

Giardiasis may be spread either directly by feces from an asymptomatic carrier or by sewage contaminating a water supply, as well as by hand-to-mouth transfer of cysts. Standard concentrations of chlorine in public

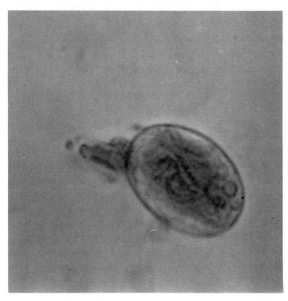

FIG. 17.3. *GIARDIA LAM-
BLIA.* IODINE-STAINED
CYST FROM STOOL

Courtesy of Elliot Scientific Corp. and Abbott Laboratories

water supplies fail to destroy giardia cysts. In the investigation of waterborne outbreaks of giardiasis, the incubation period was found to be between 1 and 4 weeks after exposure.

Precautions against spread are similar to those recommended for amebiasis, namely, sanitary disposal of feces, protection of surface water supplies against fecal contamination, and health education of families and institutionalized children. It is important to look for undiagnosed cases by microscopic examination of household members and suspected contacts. Clusters of cases should be epidemiologically investigated to determine the source of infection and the mode of transmission. If a surface water supply is involved, it should receive chemical pretreatment with sedimentation and filtration.

The treatment of choice for giardiasis is quinacrine hydrochloride (Atabrine) 100 mg t.i.d. for 5 days. It should be given with caution to patients 60 years or older and to persons of any age with a psychosis since quinicrine may cause a transitory toxic psychosis.

The New York State Department of Health Disease Control Bulletin (N.Y. State Dep. Health 1979) reported that the City of Bradford, Pa., experienced an outbreak of giardiasis in the previous several months. A total of 413 cases had been confirmed. Environmental studies implicated the city water supply and a "boil water" order was issued by the State Health Department. Additional concentrations of chlorine were added in the water supply which seemed to have solved the problem. In 1975 about 10% of the 46,000 residents of Rome, N.Y., were affected in an outbreak also attributed to contaminated water.

The Center for Disease Control reported on March 21, 1980, that outbreaks of giardiasis have been occurring throughout the country because of contamination of water supplies and that it was expected that they will continue to occur until many water supplies are improved (U.S. Dep. Health, Educ. Welfare, Cent. Dis. Control 1980). Outbreaks were reported during 1979 in California, Colorado, Oregon, Pennsylvania, Utah, and Washington.

Federal epidemiologists found that the areas where outbreaks occurred used surface water from streams, rivers, and lakes, and not well water. The principal method for the treatment of water was chlorination and did not include filtration.

Recommendation was made to officials to introduce filtration of their water supply, and to the public to boil all drinking water in order to kill the parasites.

It is believed that the source of the protozoans in some areas may have been animals, such as beavers, and in other areas probably infected humans.

BALANTIDIASIS

Another protozoan waterborne disease of the colon occasionally occurs in epidemics in areas with poor environmental sanitation. It is caused by *Balantidium coli*, a ciliated protozoan. The symptoms of the infection are somewhat similar to those of amebiasis with the feces containing blood, pus, and mucus. In severe cases there is tenderness over the colon, abdominal colic, diarrhea or constipation, anorexia, loss of weight, muscular weakness, and anemia. Its incubation period is believed to be several days.

It is transmitted by the ingestion of water contaminated with feces from infected man or hogs. It may also be acquired by hand-to-mouth transfer of feces, by raw vegetables washed with contaminated water, by soiled hands, by the association with infected swine, and by flies. The incidence of the disease in man is low as most individuals have a natural resistance to it, but it may prove serious, even fatal, to debilitated persons.

Diagnosis is made, as in the other protozoan infections, by identifying the cysts of the protozoa in the feces, or trophozoites obtained by sigmoidoscopy. Fecal examination of contacts is recommended.

Preventive measures are similar to those for amebiasis: the sanitary disposal of feces, protection of public water supplies against fecal contamination, boiling of drinking water in endemic areas, health education in personal hygiene, and handwashing. In addition, care must be taken to avoid contact with hog feces and investigation should be made of suspected hogs.

Infection may be eliminated with Diodoquin 650 mg t.i.d. for 20 days, or tetracycline 250 mg daily for 5 days.

REFERENCES

ANON. 1963. Drugs for parasitic infections. Med. Lett. Drugs Therapy 5 (23) 89–92.

BARGEN, J.A. 1951. Present day management of amebiasis. J. Am. Med. Assoc. *145*, 785.

BENENSON, A.S. 1975. Control of Communicable Diseases in Man, 12th Edition. American Public Health Association, Washington, D.C.

BENNETT, I.L., JR. 1962. Protozoan diseases. *In* Principles of Internal Medicine, Vol. 2, 4th Edition. T.R. Harrison *et al.* (Editors). Blakiston Division, McGraw-Hill Book Co., New York.

CRAUN, G.F. 1979. Waterborne giardiasis in the United States. A review. Am. J. Public Health *69*, 817.

ELSDON-DEW, R. 1968. The epidemiology of amoebiasis. Adv. Parasitol. *6*, 1.

FAUST, E.C., BEAVER, P.C. and JUNG, R.C. 1968. Animal Agents and Vectors of Human Disease. Lea and Febiger, Philadelphia.

HEALY, G.R. and GLEASON, N.N. 1969. Parasitic infections. *In* Foodborne Infections and Intoxications. H. Riemann (Editor). Academic Press, New York.

HUNTER, G.W., III, SWARTZWELDER, J.C. and CLYDE, B.F. 1976. Tropical Medicine, 5th Edition. W.B. Saunders Co., Philadelphia.

N.Y. STATE DEP. HEALTH. 1979. "Notes." N.Y. State Dep. Health Dis. Control Bull. *1* (13) 1.

REES, C.W. 1965. Problems in Amebiasis. Charles C. Thomas, Springfield, Ill.

SCHNEIERSON, S.S. 1965. Atlas of Diagnostic Microbiology. Abbott Laboratories, North Chicago.

SCHULTZ, M.G. 1975. Giardiasis. J. Am. Med. Assoc. *233*, 1384.

SHAFFER, J.G., SHLAES, W.H. and RADKE, R.A. 1965. Amebiasis. A Biomedical Problem. Charles C. Thomas, Springfield, Ill.

SHAW, P.K. *et al.* 1977. A communitywide outbreak of giardiasis with evidence of transmission by a municipal water supply. Am. Intern. Med. *87*, 426.

SULLIVAN, B.H. and BAILEY, F.N. 1951. Amebic lung abscess. Dis. Chest *20*, 84.

U.S. DEP. HEALTH, EDUC. WELFARE, CENT. DIS. CONTROL. 1980. Waterborne giardiasis. Morbidity Mortality *29* (11) 121.

WOLFE, M.S. 1978. Giardiasis. N. Engl. J. Med. *298*, 319.

18

Parasitic Foodborne and
Waterborne Diseases

A parasitic disease is one due to the presence and vital activity of an animal living on or in another animal. The unicellular organisms, *Entamoeba histolytica* and *Giardia lamblia*, and the diseases they cause have been discussed. Attention will now be directed to the multicellular parasites, namely, the helminths or worms that invade man through his digestive tract. Their identification, life cycle, mode of transmitting disease in man, the symptoms they produce, measures recommended for the prevention of spread, and treatment of the illness they cause will be described.

The parasitic diseases are no longer limited to the tropical and subtropical countries. With increased world travel and immigration of displaced persons from endemic areas, these diseases are being brought to many countries in the temperate zones. They now occur chiefly among children of underprivileged populations living under substandard sanitation. In spite of the efforts made by public health authorities in educating the public about how these infections spread and how they may be prevented, the parasitic diseases continue to occur. In many instances complete cures are often difficult to obtain. Treatment is frequently ineffective. A child with intestinal worms who has been treated and is rid of the parasites may become reinfected if poor personal hygiene, an unsanitary environment, and exposure to human excreta are not corrected.

As with the bacterial and viral foodborne and waterborne diseases, sufficient emphasis cannot be placed on the importance of the sanitary disposal of human feces, as the eggs, larvae, or adult worms are found in the excreta of infected persons. They may be spread directly when such feces contaminate a source of drinking water, or indirectly by hands soiled with feces transferring the parasites or their eggs to food. Man may also become infected by ingesting the meat of animals that harbor parasites or their larvae in their flesh, as in the case of trichinosis.

136

Man serves as a host to a number of different parasites. Among them are the various roundworms, tapeworms, and flukes (nematodes, cestodes, and trematodes). Some, like the roundworms and tapeworms, infect man directly when their eggs or larvae enter his digestive system. Others, like the flukes, require an intermediate host to complete their life cycle before they can attack man.

There are a number of drugs recommended for the treatment of the helminthic diseases, but some have serious toxic effects and must be administered with caution. When using the drugs, the manufacturer's package insert should be consulted for the drug's toxicity and side effects. In severe infestations, it is advisable to consult with a specialist in parasitic diseases.

Our efforts in deworming infected children and adults, sanitizing the environment, and educating the public have failed to eradicate the intestinal parasites. It is hoped that the time will soon come when there will be a sufficient enlistment of trained public health personnel and adequate funds made available to carry out intensive preventive programs that will result in the intestinal worms' becoming endangered and extinct species.

The following are the foodborne and waterborne diseases caused by the various helminths that are described:

Nematodes (roundworms):   Trichinosis
                           Ascariasis (roundworm disease)
                           Trichuriasis (whipworm disease)
                           Enterobiasis (pinworm disease)
                           Angiostrongyliasis (rat lungworm disease)
                           Visceral larva migrans
                           Intestinal capillariasis
                           Hepatic capillariasis

Cestodes (tapeworms):   Taeniasis (beef tapeworm disease)
                           Cysticercosis (pork tapeworm disease)
                           Hydatidosis (dog tapeworm disease)
                           Diphyllobothriasis (fish tapeworm disease)
                           Hymenolepiasis (dwarf tapeworm disease)

Trematodes (flukes):   Fasciolopsiasis (intestinal fluke disease)
                           Clonorchiasis (liver fluke disease)
                           Paragonimiasis (lung fluke disease)

TRICHINOSIS

Trichinosis is a nematode disease caused by small roundworms, *Trichinella spiralis*, commonly known as trichinae. These parasites occur most commonly in human beings, hogs, bears, cats, dogs, rats, and other carnivorous mammals.

Source of Infection

Humans usually acquire trichinosis as a result of eating infected raw or inadequately cooked pork or improperly processed pork products containing muscle tissue of swine. Hogs become infected by eating meat from carcasses of other hogs, offal from slaughterhouses, garbage containing scraps of raw pork, or infected rats. The cannibalistic rat becomes infected by devouring the carcasses of fellow rats, dogs, cats, or other animals that harbor the encysted stage of trichinae, as well as scraps of infected pork or offal. Feeding uncooked garbage to hogs, a practice still in use in some areas, is largely responsible for the propagation of trichinosis.

It is surprising that an animal that eats such repulsive food should have muscle tissue that is so delectable and appetizing. It is likewise paradoxical that meat so palatable should prove so dangerous when it is not properly cooked. However, if thoroughly cooked until the meat changes from pink to white, pork may be enjoyed with no fear of infection.

Case Report

It must be remembered that hogs are not the only animals that serve as hosts to the trichinae. A report in Morbidity and Mortality of the National Communicable Disease Center (NCDC) of the U.S. Department of Health, Education, and Welfare, Public Health Service, for April 18, 1970, reads as follows:

On January 16, 1970, samples of tongue and diaphragm examined at NCDC from a black bear killed in Pennsylvania were found infected with 110 *Trichinella spiralis* larvae per gram of tissue. The state public health veterinarian was notified, and he, in turn, investigated the source of the meat. It was learned that the bear had been shot on Nov. 28, 1969, and that the meat had been distributed among six families.

These families were contacted. Members from three of them had eaten the meat, and one family reported illnesses which were not confirmed as trichinosis. During the third week in January, the father of the ill family had eaten fried bear steak which he had shared with his three children and their friend. Three of the four children suffered sore throats and symptoms suggesting an upper respiratory infection. The fourth child had a gastrointestinal upset. The father experienced mild stomach upset and diarrhea after eating the steak, and the mother who did not taste the steak had a similar illness. All persons have recovered. Eosinophil counts on the father and the children ranged from 0−5 percent and serologic tests were negative for trichinosis.

Three of the six families who had received meat had discarded it because it "didn't look right." The mother of one of these families had thrown it away in a nearby garbage dump, located three miles from where the bear had been shot in a county where many persons come to hunt in the fall. The dump is one where bears are known to feed.

The bear meat had been examined at NCDC because Pennsylvania is one of six states participating in a study at NCDC which was begun in 1967 to determine the prevalence of trichinosis in the black bear population of the northeastern United States (MMWR, Vol. 18, No. 46).

During the course of this study five bears were found infected with *T. spiralis* larvae out of 371 examined. Two of these five bears were killed in areas where bears are known to feed on garbage; one of the bears is reported on above. It is interesting to note that some of the raw infected bear meat was disposed of in an open garbage dump where bears previously have been seen feeding on garbage. This would provide an opportunity for continued transmission of trichinosis infection.

Life Cycle

The essential phases of the life history of trichinae, which are intimately related to the various manifestations of trichinosis, are as follows: When infection occurs as a result of the ingestion of trichinous meat by a human being, the encapsulated larvae in the pork muscle tissue become freed in the stomach and migrate to the small intestine where they undergo several successive molts and emerge as sexually mature worms within 2 to 3 days (Fig. 18.1). Following copulation, the female pene-

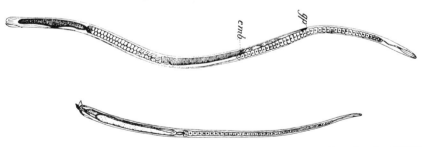

From Leuckart (1867)

FIG. 18.1. TOP—*TRICHINELLA SPIRALIS*. ADULT FEMALE SHOWING EMBRYOS *(EMB)* IN UTERUS; GENITAL OPENING *(GP)* THROUGH WHICH THE EMBRYOS ARE DISCHARGED (ENLARGED DRAWING).
BOTTOM—*TRICHINELLA SPIRALIS*. ADULT MALE (ENLARGED DRAWING).

trates deeply into the membrane that lines the intestine, and the young worms that have developed within her escape 4 or 5 days after infection.

The production of young worms continues actively for a period of about 2 weeks, after which the birth rate gradually slows down. The young worms reach the bloodstream by way of the lymph channels and are distributed by the arterial circulation to all parts of the body. They penetrate various organs and spaces in the body but achieve their full growth, as a rule, in voluntary muscles of the host. In these muscles they finally become spirally rolled and enclosed in connective tissue capsules (Fig. 18.2). If the infected subject remains alive, the capsules undergo a gradual calcification in the course of time, and sooner or later the parasites die and degenerate or else undergo a similar calcification process.

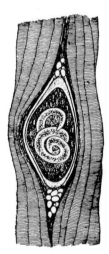

FIG. 18.2. LARVAE OF *TRICHINELLA SPIRALIS* ENCYSTED IN A PIECE OF MUSCLE (ENLARGED DRAWING)

From Leuckart (1867)

Course of the Disease

The course and gravity of trichinosis depend on the number of encysted larvae taken into the body. Slightly infected raw or improperly cooked pork will produce a mild form of the disease often passing without any special notice, whereas even a small quantity of heavily infected pork will cause an acute attack of trichinosis.

In severe infections, 3 stages of the disease may be distinguished as a rule. These stages correspond to the behavior of the parasites within the body of the infected host. In the host, they may produce musculoskeletal, gastrointestinal, cardiac, or neurological manifestations.

(1) The Stage of Ingression.—This corresponds to the development of the parasites in the intestine and the production of their brood of larvae. Gastrointestinal symptoms with nausea, vomiting, diarrhea, and severe abdominal pains may appear within several hours after the ingestion of the contaminated pork. There is also a general dullness with a feeling of weakness, twitching, tension, and pain in the muscles of the limbs, with edema (swelling) of the hands, face, and eyelids. Fever usually occurs early and may show remissions throughout the second stage.

(2) The Stage of Digression.—This stage appears within 9 to 14 days after ingestion when the larvae are distributed to the muscles by the general circulation. Severe muscular pains, especially of the flexor muscles, is manifest and the involved muscles become tense, hard, and swollen. The eyeballs become inflamed and painful on movement, showing small hemorrhages. Splinter hemorrhages occur under the fingernails due to the lodging of migrating larvae in the small blood vessels. There is profuse sweating. With the invasion of larvae in the muscles of mastication, deglutition, and respiration, there is difficulty in chewing, swallowing, breathing, and speech. These disturbances become aggravated during the fourth or fifth week after the ingestion of trichinous meat.

(3) The Stage of Regression.—This corresponds to the period of encystment of the parasites and begins 6 weeks after ingestion. The symptoms of the second stage become more pronounced. In addition, the legs, forearms, abdominal wall, and face become swollen. This is caused by acute endovascular and perivascular inflammation provoked by larvae migrating through blood vessels in those locations. Lymphadenopathy (swelling of lymph nodes) frequently appears. The patient becomes anemic and various skin eruptions appear. He is likely to develop myocarditis or pneumonia. Death due to complications such as myocarditis or encephalomeningitis may occur from the fourth to the sixth week, rarely before the second or after the seventh week. The mortality rate may be as high as 30% in some outbreaks. Those who survive may carry the encysted larvae in their muscle tissue for the rest of their lives.

Diagnosis

Although there are a number of useful diagnostic laboratory aids, early recognition of trichinosis must be made on the clinical signs, as the laboratory tests do not afford positive findings until rather late in the course of the disease. The intradermal (skin) test with *Trichinella* extract usually becomes positive on or about the seventeenth day and at times not until the fourth week. Precipitin, flocculation, and complement fixation tests become positive somewhat later, usually after the third or fourth week. Muscle biopsy, in an attempt to isolate encysted larvae, is not helpful until the third week of illness, and even then may be negative unless inflammation is heavy. Larvae may occasionally be recovered from the blood or spinal fluid, but adult parasites are very rarely found in the feces. Eosinophilia appears within 1 or 2 weeks. Eosinophils are frequently in the range of 15 to 50% of white blood cells but may rise as high as 89%. This is a valuable diagnostic aid.

Control and Prevention

No practical system of inspection of pork has as yet been devised by which persons who eat raw or imperfectly cooked pork or pork products may be protected. Even the microscopic inspection of pork for the presence of trichinae is inherently imperfect and cannot be relied on as a completely effective preventive measure, especially with lightly infected carcasses. It therefore appears that the only safe rule is to cook thoroughly all pork and its products. The housewife should remember that large pieces of pork require a much longer cooking time than small ones in order to permit the heat to penetrate the center of the meat and destroy the trichinae.

It has been demonstrated that trichinous meat may be rendered noninfectious by freezing, as exposure to $-15°C$ ($5°F$) for 2 weeks kills the *Trichinella*. Hence storage of pork in a home freezer at temperatures between $-17.8°$ and $-15°C$ ($0°$ and $5°F$) will render it fit to eat. Studies also indicate that gamma irradiation of pork with cobalt 60 kills encysted larvae. The practical commercial application of radiation of meats requires further study.

Education of the general population, especially certain ethnic groups that process their own pork products and eat them raw, must point out the danger of such customs. Investigation of a family outbreak of trichinosis revealed that they all had eaten raw sausage made at home from pork scraps. Illness is even known to have occurred among persons who had no knowledge of having eaten pork, as was the case of another family outbreak recently investigated. Hamburgers of chopped beef cooked rare were eaten by the members of the family several times during 2 weeks prior to the outbreak. The housewife usually purchased a piece of solid beef and requested the butcher to grind it. As the butcher used the same grinder for beef and pork, the remains of pork from a previous grinding admixed with the housewife's beef and contaminated it with trichinae.

Prevention in humans depends primarily on control of infection in swine. Garbage and offal fed to them should be rendered noninfectious by adequate cooking, rapid freezing, or irradiation at low dosage. The proper cooking of pork and its products to at least $65.6°C$ ($150°F$) remains the most effective prophylactic measure against trichinosis. Government inspection of pork is considered impractical and costly, affording a false sense of security.

Treatment

As for treatment, the majority of patients do not require therapy. There is no known chemotherapeutic agent that will directly attack larvae in the tissues. As diagnosis is usually not made until the migratory phase is well advanced, vermifuges to kill the parasites while still in the digestive tract are of no avail. Bed rest and symptomatic treatment with corticotropin and the corticosteroids are effective in relieving fever, edema, pain, and reducing the toxicity produced by the trichinae, as well as alleviating the allergic reaction to the parasites.

In outbreaks, it is important to make an epidemiologic study to determine the common food involved and to correct faulty practices.

ASCARIASIS

Roundworm Disease

Ascariasis is an infection of the small intestine caused by the nematode, *Ascaris lumbricoides*, the large roundworm. It is most prevalent in the Southern United States, with young children being more frequently infected than adults. Its eggs are present in the feces of infected persons. The eggs are spread by food, such as salads and other raw foods contaminated with the embryonated eggs. Water polluted by sewage containing the eggs is another vehicle of transmission. Fecal contamination of soil is also a means of spread (Fig. 18.3 and 18.4).

Life Cycle.—When the eggs are ingested, they hatch in the intestine, forming larvae that penetrate the intestinal wall and migrate to the liver and lungs through the lymphatic and circulatory systems. The larvae in the lungs ascend the bronchi, are swallowed, and pass into the intestine where they grow to maturity and mate, the female producing as many as 200,000 eggs a day. The eggs then pass out with the feces. In addition to the intestine, worms may be found in the liver, peritoneal cavity, and the appendix. Worms mature in 2 months after the ingestion of the embryonated eggs and are expelled in the feces and sometimes in the vomitus.

Symptoms of the Disease.—The symptoms of roundworm infection are variable depending on the intensity of the infestation. Patients may complain of abdominal pain, nausea, vomiting, restlessness, protrudent abdomen, skin rash, and increased appetite. In severe cases, worms may collect in sufficient number to cause fatal bowel obstruction.

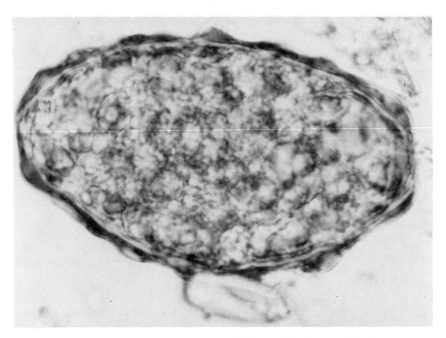

Courtesy of Elliot Scientific Corp. and Abbott Laboratories

FIG. 18.3. *ASCARIS LUMBRICOIDES*. UNSTAINED INFERTILE EGG IN FECAL SMEAR
More elongated than fertile ovum.

FIG. 18.4. *ASCARIS LUMBRICOIDES*. UN-STAINED FERTILE EGG IN FECAL SMEAR
Typical mammilated outer layer with well defined central area.

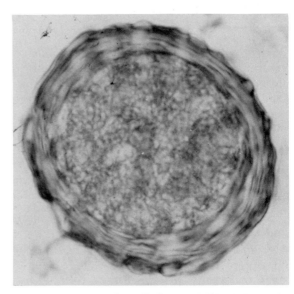

Courtesy of Elliot Scientific Corp. and Abbott Laboratories

Control and Treatment.—Infection may be prevented by the proper disposal of feces and taking measures against contamination of soil with feces, especially where children play. Children should be taught personal hygiene such as washing of hands after defecation and before eating. In endemic areas, water should be boiled and careful sanitation maintained. Ascariasis may be treated with:

(1) Piperazine citrate: Adult dose in a single dose of 3.5 g for 2 days, or
(2) Hexylresorcinol: A single dose of 1 g given on an empty stomach, followed in 2 to 4 hr with a purge of magnesium sulfate. (Hexylresorcinol is contraindicated in peptic ulcer.) The dosage for infants and children should be taken as a fraction of the adult dose as follows:

Under 7 kg (15 lb)	⅛ of adult dose
7 to 13.5 kg (15 to 30 lb)	¼ of adult dose
13.5 to 27 kg (30 to 60 lb)	½ of adult dose
Over 27 kg (60 lb)	approximately adult dose

TRICHURIASIS

Whipworm Disease

Trichuriasis is an infection of the large intestine caused by *Trichuris trichiura*, the human whipworm, a nematode 30 to 50 mm in length, that derives its name from its shape (Fig. 18.5). Cases are most prevalent in warm moist regions like the Appalachian Mountains, the lowlands of south and central Louisiana, and Puerto Rico. It is estimated that many millions of people in the world, mostly children, are infected. These persons discharging eggs in their feces make up the reservoir of infection. Eggs embryonate in contaminated soil for about 3 weeks.

Life Cycle.—Man becomes infected by ingesting embryonated eggs from contaminated hands or food (Fig. 18.6). The eggs hatch to larvae in the small intestine and pass to the colon as adult worms that attach themselves to the mucosa of the cecum and proximal colon. It takes about 90 days after ingestion before eggs are passed in the feces by the infected host.

Symptoms of Disease.—In a light infection, outside of the passage of eggs in the feces, symptoms may be absent. In the more severe infestation, there may be nausea, vomiting, diarrhea or constipation, flatulence, distention, and epigastric pain. Chronic cases have severe anemia, blood-streaked diarrhea, weight loss, and occasional prolapse of the rectum with embedded worms.

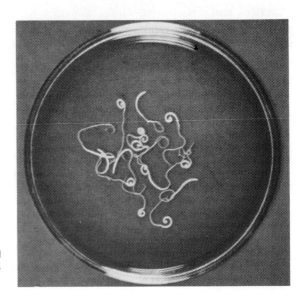

FIG. 18.5. COLLECTION
OF WHIPWORMS ON A
PETRI DISH

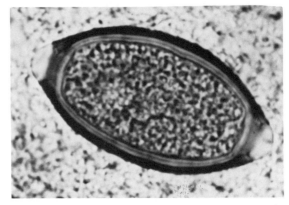

FIG. 18.6. *TRICHURIS
TRICHIURA*. UNSTAINED
EGG FROM STOOL
SPECIMEN

Courtesy of Elliot Scientific Corp. and Abbott Laboratories

Prevention and Control.—As with the other helminthic infections, cases occurring in endemic areas may be prevented by the proper disposal of feces, education of children in the proper use of toilet facilities, the washing of hands after defecation and before eating, exercising adequate sanitary measures, boiling of water, and proper cooking of food.

Treatment.—Whipworm infection may be treated with Dithiazanine iodide, 100 mg t.i.d. on first day, then increased as tolerated to 200 mg t.i.d. to a total dose of 2.7 g. Asymptomatic cases require no treatment. When the drug causes nausea, vomiting, or diarrhea, reduce the dosage or discontinue treatment. Exercise special caution in debilitated patients or those with severe renal or other disease. Watch for dehydration, depletion of electrolytes, hypotension, and acidosis, as fatality, though rare, may occur. See treatment for Ascariasis for dosage for children.

ENTEROBIASIS

Pinworm Disease

Although a relatively benign intestinal disease with mild symptoms, enterobiasis, the pinworm infection, also known as oxyuriasis, is the most common of the nematode infections. It occurs in children of grade school age, not only in the underprivileged crowded population but also in children (and their parents) in the great urban areas of America and Europe living under modern sanitary conditions.

Symptoms of the Disease.—It is caused by *Enterobius vermicularis* (Fig. 18.7), an intestinal worm about 1 cm in length that attacks humans. Symptoms are usually nonspecific with the more severe cases having anal itching, irritability, diarrhea, and anorexia. The itching is intense, causing the infected child to scratch his anal region, and often resulting in a secondary infection. The compulsive scratching plays an important role in the perpetuation of the infection in the child and its spread to his siblings, parents, and playmates.

Life Cycle.—The pinworm has a rather amazing life cycle. The gravid female worm (Fig. 18.8) migrates from the cecum to the colon and out of the anus, the exodus occurring almost precisely between 9:00 and 9:30

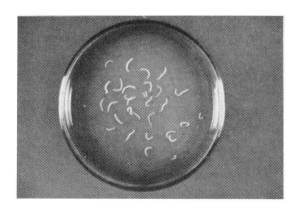

FIG. 18.7. ADULT PIN-
WORMS IN PETRI DISH

P.M., deposits over 10,000 eggs in the perianal skin, and then dies. The eggs (Fig. 18.9) remain viable for days or weeks causing the itching of the anus. The infected child scratches his anus for relief, picking up the eggs on his fingers and under his nails. The eggs are then brought to his mouth, are swallowed, hatch out, and the child thus reinfects himself. Eggs that remain in the bedclothes become airborne, contaminate the dust, and settle in the home, remaining viable in a cool moist environment for several days. Spread thus occurs not only by hand-to-mouth transfer, but through the contamination of food.

Diagnosis and Prevention.—Diagnosis may be made by observing the presence of the 1 cm long white worms occasionally on the patient's buttocks and by applying a section of Scotch® cellulose adhesive tape to the anal region in the morning and picking up the pinworm eggs for laboratory identification (Fig. 18.10 and 18.11).

The following measures are recommended for the prevention of spread and for ridding the patient and his environment of the parasites:

(1) Close-fitting underpants should be worn night and day to prevent the pinworm eggs from dropping from the host. When removed, the pants should be boiled or immediately laundered in hot water.

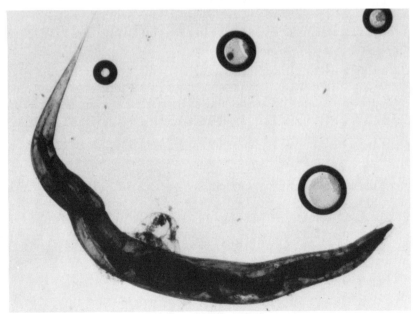

Courtesy of Elliot Scientific Corp. and Abbott Laboratories

FIG. 18.8. *ENTEROBIUS VERMICULARIS.* ADULT FEMALE WORM AS SEEN BY TRANSMITTED LIGHT
Shows oral lips, bulbous expansion of esophagus, and sharply pointed tail ("pin").

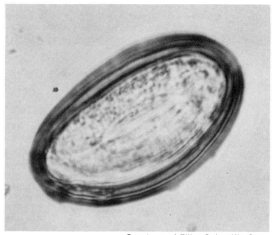

FIG. 18.9. PINWORM EGG, UNSTAINED
Elongated, ovoidal, and flattened on one side; thick, translucent shell.

Courtesy of Elliot Scientific Corp.

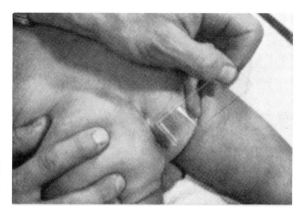

FIG. 18.10. THE CELLU-LOSE-TAPE METHOD OF OBTAINING PINWORM EGGS

(2) Daily bath and frequent trimming and cleaning of fingernails.

(3) Bed linens should be carefully removed by folding and then sterilized by boiling or laundering in very hot water.

(4) Infected individuals should not share the same bed with noninfected family members.

(5) Vacuum cleaning should be performed daily to remove some of the eggs in the house dust.

(6) Superheat the home to 35°C (95°F) or higher for a whole day as frequently as practicable to destroy the majority of eggs.

(7) The entire family should receive drug treatment when 1 or more members are infected, and the course of treatment should be repeated or prolonged if reinfection occurs.

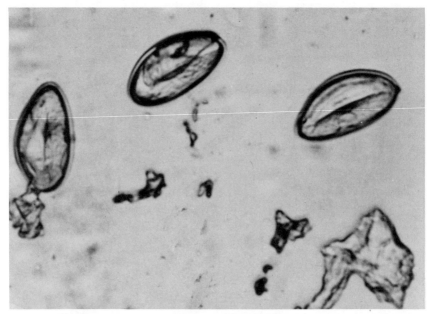

Courtesy of Elliot Scientific Corp. and Abbott Laboratories

FIG. 18.11. *ENTEROBIUS VERMICULARIS.* UNSTAINED EGGS ON ADHESIVE TAPE SWAB APPLIED TO RECTUM; MUCILAGINOUS MATERIAL OF TAPE IMPARTS THICK COATING TO SHELL

Treatment.—Treatment of pinworm infection is given as follows: Piperazine citrate, 65 mg per kg of body weight to a maximum of 2.5 g daily for 8 days; or Pyrvinium Pamoate, single dose of 5 mg per kg of body weight to a maximum of 250 mg; repeat after 2 weeks (may cause nausea and vomiting, and may turn the feces red).

ANGIOSTRONGYLIASIS

Eosinophilic Meningitis

There is a disease of the central nervous system, endemic in Eastern Asia and the South Pacific, that is caused by a nematode, *Angiostrongylus cantonensis*, the lungworm of rats. It is acquired by eating raw or undercooked fish, shrimp, snails, or land crabs infected with the larvae of the nematode. Infection in man may also occur after eating lettuce or other raw vegetables contaminated with mollusks. As in a number of other diseases, the rat is responsible for the spread of infection.

Symptoms.—The disease is a form of meningitis with severe headache, stiffness of the neck and back, areas of paresthesia, temporary facial paralysis, and low-grade fever. In some instances, the worm may enter the eyeball. Illness lasts from a few days to several months with occasional recurrences.

Diagnosis.—Diagnosis may be made by finding an increased number of white blood cells in the spinal fluid with a marked increase (25 to 100%) of eosinophils and by skin test with an antigen made from the worm.

Control.—Infection may be avoided in endemic areas by thorough cooking of all foods, particularly boiling all seafood for 3 to 5 min or freezing it at −15°C (5°F) for 24 hr to destroy the larvae. Lettuce and other greens should be carefully cleaned to eliminate any mollusks or their products that they may contain. The public should be educated in properly carrying out these precautions. Authorities in endemic areas should take measures to control and reduce the rat population.

Treatment.—Treatment is with thiabendazole (Mintezol) and should be instituted in the early stages of the disease.

VISCERAL LARVA MIGRANS

Visceral larva migrans is a disease primarily of young children. The incidence may be reduced by the passage of ordinances in communities compelling dog owners to pick up and dispose of their dog's feces in a sanitary manner. Infected cats are also capable of spreading the disease through their feces.

Source of Infection.—The disease is due to the ingestion of larvae of the nematode *Toxocara* and its migration to various organs and tissues. *Toxocara canis* is harbored by the dog, and *Toxocara cati* by the cat. Often puppies are congenitally infected while still in the uterus of the infected bitch. Cats become infected by ingesting mice that in turn have ingested ova of *Toxocara cati*.

Course of Disease.—Illness occurs in humans when *Toxocara* eggs are ingested by eating soil contaminated with infected dog or cat feces, by hand-to-mouth transmission, or by food containing the eggs. When the eggs that have embryonated while in the soil reach the intestine, they hatch and the liberated larvae penetrate the wall of the gut and migrate to the liver and lungs by the lymphatic or circulatory systems. From these organs they migrate to other organs and tissues, forming granulomatous lesions.

Symptoms depend on the invasive dose of larvae. After an incubation period of weeks or months, the infected child will develop generalized symptoms characterized by fever, a marked eosinophilia (80–90%) with an increased white cell blood count (as high as 80,000/mm^3), an enlarged liver, and an increased globulinemia. Larvae migrating to various organs such as the lungs, the eyes, and the central nervous system may cause pneumonitis (inflammation of the lungs), endophthalmitis (inflammation of the eyeball), and encephalitis (inflammation of the brain). Although symptoms may persist as long as a year or two, it is rarely a fatal disease.

Diagnosis.—Clinical diagnosis is difficult. It may be confirmed by sero-diagnostic test and by the isolation of *Toxocara* larvae on liver biopsy.

Prevention and Control.—Prevention and control of visceral larva migrans may be accomplished by preventing the contamination of soil by dogs and cats by the deep burial of their feces if passed in play areas. As children's sandboxes are often regarded by cats as a public convenience, they should be covered at night with wire netting. Puppies and kittens should be dewormed at about 3 to 6 weeks of age with piperazine, and thereafter every 6 months.

Families should be informed of the source and origin of infection, and children particularly should be prevented from eating soil. Hands should be thoroughly washed after handling soil and before eating or handling food. Infected children may be treated with diethylcarbamazine (Hetrazan).

INTESTINAL CAPILLARIASIS

An intestinal disease that is waterborne to fish and foodborne to man was first described in Manila in 1963. Four years later a severe epidemic occurred in Thailand. The disease is caused by the nematode *Capillaria philippinensis* that attacks man's small intestine causing malabsorption of food with massive protein loss, resulting in extreme emaciation. Severe and fatal cases excrete large numbers of parasites in their feces, and develop ascites (abdominal dropsy) and pleural transudate (fluid in the pleural cavity).

Fish acquire the infective larvae from other animals and man becomes infected when he ingests raw or inadequately cooked fish.

Illness may be prevented by the thorough cooking of fish or other foods from animal origin and by the sanitary disposal of feces from infected persons.

HEPATIC CAPILLARIASIS

There is another form of capillariasis that commonly occurs in rats and in a number of mammals but only rarely in man. Human cases have been reported in North America, Mexico, Brazil, Hawaii, Turkey, and India.

Life Cycle.—The disease is due to the nematode *Capillaria hepatica*. The adult worms remain in the liver of the infected animal where they generate eggs. When the animal host dies, the liver decomposes, and the eggs may contaminate the soil and a water source. If the eggs are eaten by another animal, they form larvae that penetrate the gut, enter the portal system, and are filtered out in the liver. Should the animal be one that serves as food for humans and its liver is eaten, or if other contaminated food or water is ingested, the life cycle of the parasite is repeated in man resulting in a severe form of hepatitis with marked ascites, weight loss, and emaciation often proving fatal.

As in the other helminthic diseases, there is an increased eosinophilia, and eggs of the parasites may be isolated from the patient's feces.

The protection of water supplies and of foods contaminated with soil may serve as preventive measures.

TAENIASIS AND CYSTICERCOSIS

Beef and Pork Tapeworm Diseases

Taeniasis is an infection with the adult stage of the beef tapeworm, *Taenia saginatum*. Infection with the adult or larval stage of the pork tapeworm, *Taenia solium*, is referred to as cysticercosis. The latter is the more serious of the tapeworm infections as it is a somatic disease involving not only the digestive tract but also other organs and tissues in which encystment occurs.

Courses of the Diseases.—When the larvae of *T. saginata* (the beef tapeworm), present in infected raw or rare beef are ingested, they hatch in the small intestine and the adult worm develops. Symptoms of taeniasis (beef tapeworm infection) are variable. The patient may be asymptomatic, or he may have digestive disturbances, abdominal pain, anorexia, nervousness, insomnia, and loss of weight. Taeniasis is considered to be a nonfatal disease.

On the other hand, when eggs of *T. solium* (the pork tapeworm) are swallowed with raw or lightly cooked pork, they hatch in the small intestine and larval forms (cysticerci) develop in the subcutaneous tissues, striated muscle, and other tissues, including the heart, eyes, and central nervous system. Such infections often prove fatal.

Diagnosis.—The adult tapeworm in the intestine throws off distal segments (proglottids) each containing a gravid uterus. Diagnosis may be made by identifying these segments of the worm or of the eggs in the feces (Fig. 18.12). Eggs are picked up by using an adhesive cellulose tape swab. Subcutaneous or visceral cysticerci, if present, may be excised and the larvae identified.

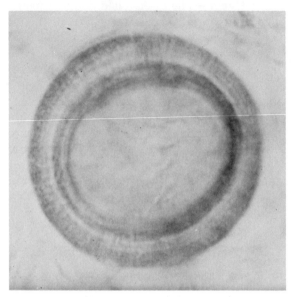

FIG. 18.12. *TAENIA* SPE-
CIES. UNSTAINED EGG
IN STOOL SPECIMEN.
HOOKLETS IN EMBRYO
FAINTLY VISIBLE

Courtesy of Elliot Scientific Corp. and Abbott Laboratories

Reservoir of Infection.—As with the other parasitic diseases, infected man discharging eggs of the parasite in his feces serves as the reservoir of infection. Cattle and swine become infected by eggs in human feces contaminating the soil, feed, or water. Infection is spread to other humans who eat the raw or inadequately cooked meat of these animals. Man may harbor the adult worm in his intestine for as long as 30 to 40 years, all the while disseminating the eggs in the environment.

Prevention.—Human cysticercosis and taeniasis may be prevented by:

(1) Immediate treatment of infected persons until the scolex (head of the tapeworm) that is hooked to the mucous membrane of the intestine is expelled in the feces.
(2) Education of the public in rural areas in the sanitary disposal of feces and preventing their contamination of the soil or water supply.
(3) The thorough cooking of meats.
(4) Adequate inspection of carcasses of cattle and swine, and condemnation of those found to be infected.
(5) Avoidance of use of sewage effluent for pasture irrigation.
(6) Not permitting swine access to latrines or to human feces.
(7) Exclusion of infected persons from preparing or serving food.
(8) Washing of hands after defecation and before eating.

Treatment.—The drugs recommended for the treatment of tapeworm infection are:

(1) Quinacrine hydrochloride (Atabrine): 4 doses of 200 mg 10 min apart; 600 mg sodium bicarbonate with each dose. Give with caution to patients over 60 years old or those with a history of psychosis at any age, as it may cause a transitory toxic psychosis.

(2) Oleoresin of aspidium: 4 to 8 g plus 8 g of acacia in water. Give one-half of the dose early in the morning and the rest 1 hr later; or give a single dose by duodenal tube in order to prevent vomiting.

HYDATIDOSIS

Dog Tapeworm Disease

In many towns and cities in the United States, the law requires that when a dog relieves himself while being walked, his master is required to pick up his pet's feces and dispose of them in a sanitary manner. Scoops and plastic bags are available for that unpleasant task. Should the dog be harboring *Salmonella* or an intestinal parasite, such as tapeworm, his master exposes himself to infection unless he handles the feces carefully and does not soil his hands. Fortunately, hydatidosis or dog tapeworm disease is relatively rare in this country, occurring primarily in the Middle East, Central Europe, Australia, and South America.

Reservoir of Infection.—The dog tapeworms, *Echinococcus granulosus* and *E. multilocularis*, are found not only in dogs but also in other members of the Canidae family such as wolves, dingoes, and foxes. Infective eggs are excreted in the feces of these animals and, in the case of the dog, are present on his fur and harness and in the living environment of man.

Forms of Hydatidosis.—*Unilocular Echinococcosis or Hydatid Disease.*—There are 2 forms of hydatidosis. One is the disease caused by *E. granulosus*, known as unilocular echinococcosis or hydatid disease. It is transmitted to man by the ingestion of infective eggs in foods or water contaminated with the feces of infected animals, by hand-to-mouth transfer of dog's feces or by objects soiled with feces. Dogs become infected by eating hydatid cysts in the viscera of dead herbivorous animals. They begin to shed eggs of the parasite in their feces about 6 weeks after such ingestion. The eggs are resistant and may survive for years in soil or in households. When the eggs are ingested by man, they hatch in the intestine and the larvae migrate to various organs such as the liver, lungs, and occasionally the kidneys, heart, bone, thyroid, and the central nervous system, where they form cysts of various sizes.

Symptoms depend on the location and size of the cysts. In some organs no symptoms occur if the cysts are small, but if they are excessive in size or are in vital organs, they may cause severe symptoms and death. The disease is not directly transmitted from man to man as man does not harbor the adult worm.

Alveolar Hydatid Disease.—The other form of dog tapeworm disease is the alveolar hydatid disease caused by *E. multilocularis.* This type of tapeworm is also found in foxes and wolves. It is similarly spread to man by the ingestion and hand-to-mouth transfer of infective eggs from the dog's feces, his fur, or his environment.

Diagnosis.—Diagnosis of alveolar hydatidosis may be confirmed by microscopic examination of sputum, vomitus, urine, and feces, or of discharges from a ruptured cyst or a sinus, for the presence of hooklets, scolices (heads of hookworms), and cyst membrane. Other aids are complement fixation, indirect hemagglutination, latex flocculation, and intradermal tests as well as the examination of cyst tissues obtained surgically.

Control.—To control the spread of hydatidosis, it is necessary to prevent dogs from having access to uncooked viscera of slaughtered animals that may have hydatid cysts. In endemic areas, infected dogs should be licensed and their numbers reduced. Children and adults in such areas should be educated to the dangers of close association with dogs and the need for controlled slaughtering of animals. Dead animals should be incinerated or deeply buried.

Treatment.—There is no specific treatment for dog tapeworm disease. Often the surgical removal of isolated cysts may prove curative.

DIPHYLLOBOTHRIASIS

Fish Tapeworm Disease

Infection with the fish tapeworm, *Diphyllobothrium latum,* also known as the broad tapeworm, is a nonfatal disease of long duration, often with trivial or absent symptoms. It occurs in persons eating uncooked, freshwater fish from midwestern or Canadian lakes.

Life Cycle.—Infected man and other fish-eating mammals, such as dog or bear, discharge their feces containing tapeworm sections (proglottids) and eggs into bodies of fresh water (Fig. 18.13). There the eggs mature, hatch, and infect minute freshwater crustacea (copepods) that serve as the first intermediate host. The infected copepods are ingested by fish, the second intermediate host. In the fish, the worms infest the fish's flesh and roe and change into the form infective to man.

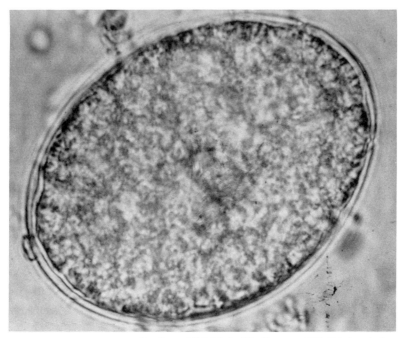

Courtesy of Elliot Scientific Corp. and Abbott Laboratories

FIG. 18.13. *DIPHYLLOBOTHRIUM LATUM*. UNSTAINED OPERCULATED EGG IN STOOL

Moderately thick shell; operculum faintly visible; a knob–like thickening is on side opposite operculum.

Symptoms.—Symptoms of fish tapeworm disease are vague. Infected persons may complain of abdominal pain, weakness, loss of weight, and anemia. They may continue to disseminate the eggs into the environment for several years. Diagnosis is made by the identification of proglottids or eggs of the tapeworm in the feces.

Control.—Spread may be controlled by: (1) education of the public in the life cycle of the parasite; (2) proper sanitary measures and handwashing; (3) prevention of stream and lake pollution with human feces by adequate sewerage; (4) thorough cooking of all freshwater fish; (5) freezing of fish for 24 hr at −10°C.

Treatment.—Treatment is identical to that for taeniasis (beef tapeworm disease) (see page 153).

HYMENOLEPIASIS

Dwarf Tapeworm Disease

A type of tapeworm that is more common in children than adults is the dwarf tapeworm known as *Hymenolepis nana*. Man and rodents serve as the reservoir of infection. With ova present in the feces of infected persons (Fig. 18.14), transmission occurs by the ingestion of food contaminated with such feces. It may also be spread by direct contact and by hand-to-mouth route.

The incubation period is about 2 months. Infected persons undergo irritation of the intestine and complain of abdominal pain and diarrhea.

As in the other helminthic infections, spread may be prevented by the sanitary disposal of the excreta of infected persons, by personal hygiene including handwashing after defecation and before eating or the handling of food eaten by other persons, by food sanitation, and by rodent control.

Treatment is with quinacrine hydrochloride (Atabrine): 4 doses of 200 mg 10 min apart, and 600 mg sodium bicarbonate with each dose; repeat in 1 or 2 weeks if necessary.

FASCIOLOPSIASIS

Intestinal Fluke Disease

The infective agent for this trematode disease is *Fasciolopis buski*, a large fluke that invades the small intestine causing abdominal pain,

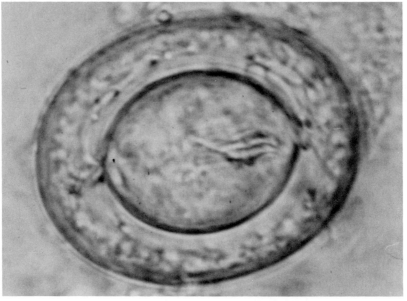

Courtesy of Elliot Scientific Corp. and Abbott Laboratories

FIG. 18.14. *HYMENOLEPIS NANA.* UNSTAINED EGG FROM STOOL
Embryo with 6 hooklets (all not visible); polar filaments in inner shell.

vomiting, anorexia, diarrhea with greenish feces alternating with constipation, and swelling of the face, abdominal wall, and limbs. Blood study
reveals anemia with eosinophilia. Intestinal obstruction may be caused
by an accumulation of large numbers of flukes. The disease is widely
distributed in the Orient.

Life Cycle.—Infected man, dog, or pig excretes the flukes or their eggs
in its feces, occasionally vomiting the worms. Water may thus become
contaminated. In the water, eggs from the infected feces develop into
embryos of the fluke (miracidia), hatch, and penetrate snails, the intermediate host. In the snails, free-swimming larvae (cercariae) develop.
They are liberated and encyst on aquatic edible plants. Man and other
mammals become infected by eating the plants uncooked, with illness
occurring 1 to 2 months after ingestion.

Diagnosis.—Diagnosis is made by finding flukes or their characteristic
eggs in the feces. The flukes measure 20 to 75 mm in length, 8 to 20 mm
in width, and 0.5 to 3 mm in thickness.

Prevention.—Infection may be prevented by educating the public in
endemic areas to destroy the cercariae on the plants such as roots of
lotus, water chestnuts, bamboo, and caltrops, by either cooking them or
else dipping them in boiling water before eating. Cercariae may also be
destroyed by drying the plants. As in the other intestinal infections,
sanitary disposal of feces and avoiding the use of night soil are recommended. The destruction of the snails, if practical, is another control
measure.

Treatment.—The drugs that are reasonably effective in the treatment
of intestinal fluke disease are:

(1) Tetrachlorethylene: A single dose of 0.12 ml/kg of body weight in
    gelatin capsules (not more than 5 ml); it may cause nausea and
    inebriation, and rarely loss of consciousness. The patient should be
    kept at rest after the drug is administered. No alcohol should be
    taken before or for 24 hr after the drug.
(2) Hexylresorcinol: 1 g as a single dose given on an empty stomach,
    followed in 2 to 4 hr with a purge of magnesium sulfate. It is
    contra-indicated in peptic ulcer.

CLONORCHIASIS

Liver Fluke Disease

Clonorchiasis is also known as the Chinese liver fluke disease because it
is a trematode disease of the bile ducts that occurs in the Far East. With

the migration of Koreans and Vietnamese into the United States, the disease is expected to make its appearance here.

Life Cycle.—Man becomes infected by eating raw or partly-cooked freshwater fish that harbor *Clonorchis sinensis*, the Asiatic liver fluke. In the intestine, the larvae are set free from the ingested cysts and migrate via the bile ducts to the biliary radicles (small liver ducts). The eggs deposited in the bile ducts contain developed embryos (miracidiae) and are evacuated in the feces (Fig. 18.15). When the feces pollute a fresh body of water, the eggs are ingested by a susceptible snail (the first intermediary host), in which they hatch and form cercariae (free-swimming larvae). The larvae emerge in the water, and penetrate and encyst in the muscle tissue of fish (the second intermediate host) on the underside of the scales. Man, dog, cat, or pig on eating the fish becomes infected and in time discharges the fluke eggs in its feces. The complete life cycle from man to man requires about 3 months and infected persons may continue to shed eggs for as long as 30 years.

Symptoms.—In mild infections, symptoms may be minimal with anorexia and sensation of abdominal pressure. In the chronic cases, flukes irritating the bile ducts may cause obstruction to the flow of bile, resulting in enlargement and tenderness of the liver, ascites (abdominal dropsy), and cirrhosis.

Diagnosis.—Diagnosis, as with the other helminthic diseases, is made by the presence of eggs of the flukes in the feces. Flukes may also be obtained on duodenal drainage. Differential blood count reveals an eosinophilia.

Control.—Spread may be controlled through treatment of infected persons, education of the public in the life cycle of the parasite, thorough cooking of freshwater fish, and the boiling of drinking water in endemic areas. The use of night soil as fertilizer in fish ponds should be abandoned. If its use is continued, 1 part of 0.7% solution of ammonium sulfate should be added to 10 parts of feces to kill the miracidiae in the eggs within 30 min.

Treatment.—Treatment is with chloroquine diphosphate, 250 mg t.i.d. for 6 weeks. This may not produce a cure, but it may cause a temporary suppression of ova. Chloroquine may cause nausea and vomiting, nervousness, insomnia, headache, and blurring of vision, but evidently not irreversible eye changes such as occur in long-term use.

Fascioliasis—Sheep Liver Fluke Disease

Mention may be made here of fascioliasis, the sheep liver fluke disease caused by *Fasciola hepatica* that is transmitted to man by the ingestion

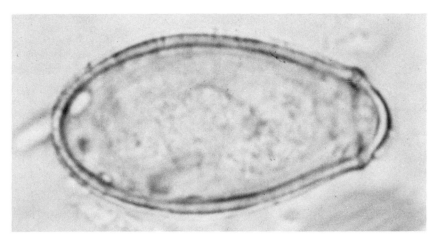

Courtesy of Elliot Scientific Corp. and Abbott Laboratories

FIG. 18.15. *CLONORCHIS SINENSIS*. UNSTAINED OPERCULATED EGG FROM STOOL
Pyriform shape and typical convex operculum; moderately thick wall.

of rare or poorly cooked liver of sheep, cattle, or other ruminants. The
disease occurs in South America, the Caribbean region and in parts of the
United States. The drug of choice for its treatment is emetine hydrochloride given as recommended for the treatment of lung fluke infection (see
following section).

PARAGONIMIASIS

Lung Fluke Disease

Lung fluke disease is a trematode infection that is endemic in the
continents of South America, Asia, and Africa. It is caused by the flukes
Paragonimus ringeri, *P. westermani*, and *P. kellicotti*. The eggs of the
flukes are found in the sputum and feces of infected persons as well as in
pig, dog, wolf, and rat. The eggs gain entrance with feces into fresh water
where the larvae hatch and penetrate into freshwater snails in which
they undergo further development into cercariae. These are released into
the water and penetrate and encyst in freshwater crustacea (crabs and
crayfish).

Life Cycle.—When infected crustacea are eaten raw or only partially
cooked, the larvae emerge in the duodenum, penetrate the intestinal wall,
and migrate through the tissues, encysting in pairs and developing into
egg-producing adults. Worms frequently mature in the lungs or other
organs such as lymph nodes, the gastrointestinal tract, and the brain.

The eggs leave the host in the sputum and feces, and may continue to do so for as long as 20 years.

Symptoms.—Symptoms consist of diarrhea, dull pains, and a chronic cough, often with hemoptysis. As in other chronic pulmonary diseases, clubbing of the fingers may occur.

Prevention.—Infection may be prevented in endemic areas through: (1) education of the public of the life cycle of the flukes; (2) sanitary disposal of sputum and feces; (3) thorough cooking of freshwater crabs and crayfish; (4) boiling of drinking water; (5) destruction of snails with molluscacides.

Treatment.—The drugs recommended for the treatment of lung fluke disease are:

(1) Emetine hydrochloride: 1 mg per kg of body weight (maximum 65 mg) daily, subcutaneously, or intramuscularly for 10 to 12 days depending on ova found in sputum. Patients receiving emetine should remain sedentary for several weeks after the drug is given because of its toxic effect on the heart.

(2) Chloroquine diphosphate: 250 mg b.i.d. for 6 weeks; may cause nausea and vomiting, nervousness, insomnia, headache, and blurring of vision.

REFERENCES

ANON. 1963. Drugs for parasitic infections. Med. Lett. Drugs Therapeutics 5 (126) 89–92.

BECK, J.W., SEAVEBRA, D., ANTELL, G.J. and TEJEIRO, B. 1959. The treatment of pinworm infection in humans (enterobiasis) with pyrvinium chloride and pyrvinium pamoate. Am. J. Trop. Med. Hyg. 8, 349.

BENENSON, A.S. 1975. Control of Communicable Diseases in Man, 12th Edition. American Public Health Association,Washington, D.C.

BUMBALO, T.S. 1961. Parasitic infections in children. N.Y. State J. Med. 61, 1843.

BUMBALO, T.S., PLUMMER, L.I. and WARNER, J.R. 1958. The treatment of enterobiasis in children. Am. J. Trop. Med. Hyg. 7, 212.

CECIL, R.L. and LOEB, R.F. 1959. A Textbook of Medicine, 10th Edition. W.B. Saunders Co., Philadelphia.

CRAIG, C.F. and FAUST, E.C. 1964. Clinical Parasitology, 7th Edition. Lea and Febiger, Philadelphia.

DUGUID, I.M. 1961. Chronic endophthalmitis due to toxocara. Br. J. Ophthalmol. 45, 705.

FAUST, E.C., BEAVER, P.C. and JUNG, R.C. 1968. Animal Agents and Vectors of Human Disease. Lea and Febiger, Philadelphia.

GOULD, S.E. 1970. Trichinosis in Man and Animals. Charles C. Thomas, Springfield, Ill.

GOULD, S.E., GOMBERG, H.J. and BETHELL, F.H. 1954. Control of trichinosis by gamma irradiation of pork. J. Am. Med. Assoc. 154, 653.

HEALY, G.R. and GLEASON, N.N. 1969. Parasitic infections. In Foodborne Infections and Intoxications. H. Reimann (Editor). Academic Press, New York.

HOLT, E.L., JR., McINTOSH, H. and BARNETT, H.L. 1962. Pediatrics, 13th Edition. Appleton-Century-Crofts, New York.

HUNTER, G.W., III, SWARTZWELDER, J.C. and CLYDE, D.F. 1976. Tropical Medicine, 5th Edition. W.B. Saunders Co., Philadelphia.

JUNG, R.C. and FAUST, E.C. 1956. The treatment of intestinal parasitic infections. AMA Arch. Internal Med. 98, 495.

KEAN, B.H. 1960. Modern treatment of common intestinal parasitic diseases. Postgrad. Med. 28, 35.

LEUCKART, R. 1867. Trichinosis. Cited in U.S. DEP. AGRIC. 1946. Trichinosis—A disease caused by eating raw pork. U.S. Dep. Agric. Leafl. 34.

NELSON, W.E. 1964. Textbook of Pediatrics, 8th Edition. W.B. Saunders Co., Philadelphia.

PAWLOWSKI, Z. and SCHULTZ, M.G. 1972. Taeniasis and cysticercosis (Taenia saginata). Adv. Parasitol. 10, 269.

RODRIGUES, V.T. et al. 1961. Treatment of oxyuriasis with a single dose of pyrvinium pamoate (Povan); preliminary note. J. Podiat. (Rio) 25, 324. Index Medicus 2 (2) 490.

ROYER, A. and BERDNIKOFF, K., 1962. Pinworm infection in children: The problem and its treatment. Can. Med. Assoc. J. 86, 60.

SCHNEIERSON, S.S. 1965. Atlas of Diagnostic Microbiology. Abbott Laboratories, North Chicago.

TARTAKOW, I.J. 1977. Casebook of a medical detective: A review of interesting cases. Nassau County Med. Cent. 4 (2) 65—73.

U.S. DEP. HEALTH, EDUC. WELFARE, PUBLIC HEALTH SERV. 1970. Trichinosis in bears. Morbidity Mortality 19 (15) 150.

VANDERZANT, C. and NICKERSON, R. 1969. A microbial examination of muscle tissue of beef, pork, and lamb carcasses. J. Milk Food Technol. 32, 357.

WRIGHT, W.H. 1955. Current status of parasitic diseases. Public Health Rep. 70, 966.

YOKOGAWA, M. 1969. Paragonimus and paragonimiasis. Adv. Parasitol. 7, 375.

19

Fungus Poisoning

Fungi consist of a group of saprophytic and parasitic lower plants that lack chlorophyll. They obtain nourishment osmotically from the dissolved products of organic breakdown and decay. Included among the fungi are molds, rusts, mildew, smuts, yeast, and mushrooms. Some fungi are capable of attacking various tissues and organs of the human body such as skin, scalp, nails, the mouth, lungs, and vagina. Others are poisonous when ingested. Discussion will be limited to the latter group.

MUSHROOM POISONING

Mycetismus

The 60-year-old man and his wife had been admitted to the hospital in a comatose condition. Their son had told the resident physician at the hospital that his parents had told him that they had gathered a quantity of wild mushrooms in the woods and had cooked and eaten them. They had become ill about 3 hr later. Both improved after gastric lavage was performed and atropine administered.

When interviewed, the male patient stated that he was surprised that the mushrooms had proved poisonous as he had had considerable experience in gathering mushrooms in Italy. He said that he knew what poisonous mushrooms looked like and that he even had made the test that distinguishes poisonous from edible mushrooms. When asked what the test was, he explained that it consists of placing a silver coin in the pot in which the mushrooms are being cooked: if the coin becomes tarnished, then the mushrooms are poisonous. As the coin had remained unchanged, he had concluded that the mushrooms were safe to eat. It appears that both his expertise as a mycetophile (mushroom lover) was wanting and his test was unreliable as some poisonous mushrooms when cooked do not give off enough sulfur to tarnish silver.

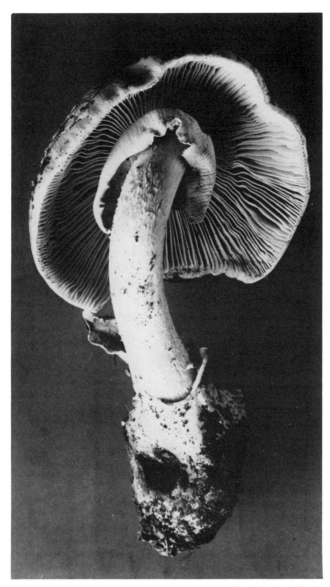

From Charles (1953)

FIG. 19.1. *AMANITA PHALLOIDES*, "DEATH CUP" (POISONOUS)
In the death cup, the color of the cap ranges from white or
lemon to olive or brownish. It is the most dangerous of all
mushrooms. It is widely distributed and of very common occurrence and may be found growing in woods or cultivated land
from spring until late autumn.

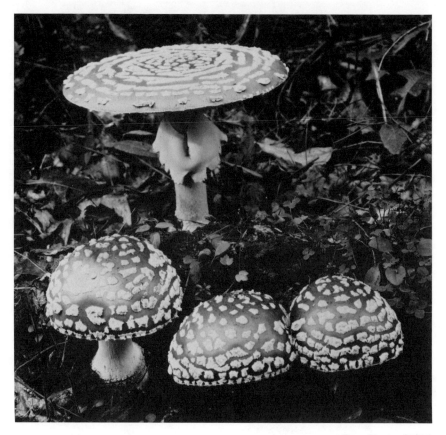

From Charles (1953)

FIG. 19.2. *AMANITA MUSCARIA*, "FLY AGARIC" (POISONOUS)
In the fly agaric, the color of the cap ranges from yellow to orange or blood red, and the remnants of the volva remain as whitish scales on the cap. The veil persists as a large, torn ring about the upper part of the stem. This species may be found during the summer and fall, singly or in small patches, or of considerable size. The color is an exceedingly variable character, being brighter in young plants and fading as they mature. It is a very poisonous species and is responsible for many deaths and numerous cases of severe poisoning.

There are a number of wild poisonous mushrooms that grow from the spring to autumn in the woods, by the roadside, and even on cultivated land. The most common belong to the *Amanita* genus, *Amanita phalloides*, also known as "death cup," and *Amanita muscaria*, referred to as "fly agaric."

The risk in eating these mushrooms may be materially reduced by the ability to recognize them, although their identification is a matter for the trained mycologist. V.K. Charles (1953) in a U.S. Department of Agriculture circular gives an excellent description of these fungi as follows:

In the death cup the color of the cap ranges from white or lemon to olive or brownish. It is broadly bell-shaped or oval and finally expanded, smooth or with patches of scales. In most weather it is very sticky. The gills are free and white and the stem mostly smooth and bulbous, surrounded by a large cup-shaped volva (a membranous sac about the base of the stipe or stem). The ring is large, white and reflexed . . . . In the fly agaric the color of the cap ranges from yellow to orange or blood red, and the remnants of the volva remain as whitish scales on the cap. The veil persists as a large torn ring about the upper part of the stem, which is white and enlarged at the base and usually marked by scaly ridges or incomplete rings.

Poisoning with *A. phalloides* is caused by alpha, beta, and gamma amanitine, a heat-stable peptide. Cooking, therefore, fails to destroy the poison that is so potent that the ingestion of only 2 or 3 such mushrooms may prove fatal within 48 hr. The onset of illness is from several minutes to 6 hr with abdominal pain, blood-tinged vomitus, and diarrhea, extreme dehydration, salivation, excessive thirst, damage of the liver resulting in jaundice, and damage of the central nervous system with confusion, collapse, and coma. The mortality rate is from 50 to 90% if untreated.

The toxin responsible for poisoning after ingesting *A. muscaria* is muscarine, an alkaloid that acts like pilocarpine on smooth muscles of the pupils and on the cells of glands of external secretion. It is somewhat less toxic than amanitine but causes comparable symptoms. The onset is from a few minutes to 2 hr.

Some lesser known poisonous mushrooms, other than those of the *Amanita* genus that should be avoided, are: *Galerina venenata, Helvella esculenta, Lactarius vellereus*, and *Lepiota morgani*. Alcoholics in particular should be wary of *Coprinus atramentarius*, also known as "inky cap," as it contains disulfiran, a toxin that inhibits the absorption of alcohol, causing violent illness in such persons.

Treatment for mushroom poisoning consists of emptying the patient's stomach as soon as possible by gastric lavage and prompt intravenous administration of atropine in a larger than usual dose (0.02 mg/kg body weight). It is necessary to restore fluids and electrolytes if vomiting or diarrhea is present. Hemodialysis (artificial kidney) may be used in severe cases to remove uremic and other toxic constituents in the blood. If treatment is prompt, the prognosis is favorable. If the patient is untreated, death may be imminent.

ERGOTISM

During the Middle Ages, there occurred in various parts of Europe epidemics of a disease characterized by an excruciating burning sensation followed by gangrene of the extremities and other parts of the body. It was known as St. Anthony's fire, named after the saint's martyrdom. In time it was found to be caused by ergot *(Claviceps purpurea)*, a highly toxic fungus that grows on rye and other grains used in the making of bread. This disease is not altogether ancient as a similar outbreak occurred as recently as 1951 in France.

Ergot is a sclerotium of *C. purpurea*, a horny elongated blackish-purple mass with a peculiar disagreeable odor, that replaces the grain of rye that it parasitizes. When ingested in bread, it causes contractions of the muscular coat of the arteries, cutting off the circulation to the extremities and resulting in gangrene of the fingers and toes, and occasionally the ears and nose. In severe cases, neurologic symptoms such as convulsions and hallucinations may occur, sometimes resulting in death.

Preceding the onset of the gangrene, patients complain of weakness, headache, and convulsive depression, and there is usually anesthesia, tingling, pains, cramps, and spasmodic movement of muscles with gradual blood stasis. The onset is insidious, occurring after the ingestion of several meals of diseased bread or meal.

Because of its ability to contract involuntary muscle, extracts of ergot or derivatives such as ergotine tartrate and ergonovine are used medically as peripheral vascular constrictors to promote the rapidity of labor and in certain forms of uterine bleeding to contract the uterus.

Ergotism in the general public may be prevented by bakers avoiding the use of diseased rye and by processors of meals likewise discarding ergot-infested grain.

In the treatment of ergotism, arterial spasm may be combatted by amylnitrite 0.3 ml by inhalation, nitroglycerin 0.4 mg sublingually, or papaverine 30 to 60 mg intramuscularly or intravenously.

MOLD POISONING

Mold is a growth of minute fungi usually found on dead or decaying vegetable or animal matter, and it usually appears as a downy or furry coating. All foods may be affected by mold if exposed to moisture and temperature favorable for its growth.

There are various types of mold. Some are harmless, and some are desirable such as the greenish-blue mold that flavors Camembert and blue cheeses. Some are beneficial, such as *Penicillium notatum*, and others produce poisonous chemicals or mycotoxins that may contaminate food. When ingested, mycotoxins can damage the liver, brain, bones, or nerves, or may interfere with the coagulation property of blood.

Aspergillus flavus, a common mold that grows on corn, figs, grain, sorghum, nuts, and peanuts, produces aflatoxin, a mycotoxin that causes

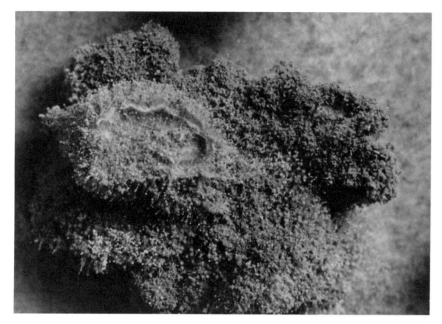

Courtesy of Food and Drug Administration

FIG. 19.3. THESE WALNUT MEATS SHOW A HEAVY CONTAMINATION BY *ASPER-GILLUS FLAVUS*, THE MOLD SPECIES WHICH PRODUCES AFLATOXIN, GROWN UN-DER IDEAL CONDITIONS IN THE LABORATORY

cancer of the liver in laboratory animals. U.S. Federal Food and Drug Administration prohibits the marketing of peanuts and peanut products that contain more than 15 parts of aflatoxin per billion. Even though industries handling such commodities are self-regulatory, FDA inspectors periodically check their products to ascertain that they do not contain more than the maximum quantity of aflatoxin. The lot of peanuts found to be highly contaminated is used for the production of peanut oil, as the refining processes eliminate all traces of aflatoxin. If the peanut meal by-product from this process is contaminated, it is used only for fertilizer. In some parts of Asia and Africa where foods with high concentration of aflatoxin are consumed, the incidence of liver cancer is relatively high.

Industry prevents mold from forming on nuts and other products by proper drying and storage of crops under adequate moisture and humidity. Consumers should discard any food showing evidence of contamination with mold. Trimming off the moldy parts of foods and eating the rest is not safe as the roots of the mold may still be present in the portion ingested.

In rice-eating countries like Japan, "yellowed rice," which is rice contaminated with certain species of *Penicillium* mold, is strongly suspected of causing cirrhosis and carcinoma of the liver as demonstrated by livestock and experimental animal feedings. In the United States, corn similarly contaminated brought about acute hepatotoxic hemorrhagic syndrome when administered to various laboratory animals including the dog.

Roquefort, Camembert, and blue cheeses are veined with mold similar to those that produce penicillin. They are perfectly safe to eat, but other cheeses that are not expected to be moldy, if they are moldy, should be avoided.

There are some strains of mold previously used in the manufacturing of cheese that have now been found to produce mycotoxin.

As mold spores are present in the air, they may also be present in the refrigerator as evidenced by the small black spots that sometimes are seen on refrigerated food. It is therefore necessary to periodically wash and dry the interior of the refrigerator to prevent the growth of mold on stored food. So, if you hear someone say, "A little mold won't hurt you," don't believe it.

REFERENCES

ALEXOPOULOS, C.J. 1967. Introductory Mycology. John Wiley & Sons, New York.

BARGER, G. 1931. Ergot and Ergotism. Gurney and Jackson, London.

BILAY, V.I. 1960. Mycotoxicoses of Man and Agricultural Animals. Office of Technical Serv., U.S. Dep. Commerce, Washington, D.C. (English translation)

CANN, H.M. and VERHULST, H. 1961. Mushroom poisoning. Am. J. Dis. Child. *101*, 128.

CHARLES, V.K. 1953. Some common mushrooms and how to know them (revised). U.S. Dep. Agric. Circ. *143*.

COOK, C.D. and HAGGERTY, R.J. 1960. Mycetismus. N. Engl. J. Med. *262*, 832.

FARGACS, J. 1962. Mycotoxicoses—The neglected diseases. Foodstuffs *34* (18) 124.

GROSSMAN, C.M. and MALBIN, B. 1954. Mushroom poisoning: A review of the literature and report of two cases caused by a previously undescribed species. Am. Internal Med. *40*, 249.

HEENAN, J. 1974. Please don't eat the mold. U.S. Public Health Serv., U.S. Dep. Health, Educ. Welfare (FDA) *75-2028*. U.S. Govt. Printing Off., Washington, D.C.

JARVIS, B. 1971. Factors affecting the production of mycotoxin. J. Appl. Bacteriol. *34*, 199.

LARKIN, T. 1975. Natural poisons in food. U.S. Public Health Serv., U.S. Dep. Health, Educ. Welfare (FDA) 76–2009. U.S. Govt. Printing Off., Washington, D.C.

LEMKE, P.A. and NASH, C.H. 1974. Fungal viruses. Bacteriol. Rev. 38, 29.

LOCKETT, S. 1957. Clinical Toxicology. C.V. Mosby Co., St. Louis.

NEWBERNE, P.M. 1974. The new world of mycotoxins—animal and human health. Clin. Toxicol. 7, 161.

SCHINDLER, A.F. et al. 1974. Mycotoxin produced by fungi isolated from inshell pecans. J. Food Sci. 39, 213.

STOLOFF, L. 1976. Report on mycotoxins. J. Assoc. Off. Anal. Chem. 59, 317.

TYLER, W.E., JR. 1963. Poisonous mushrooms. Prog. Chem. Toxicol. 1, 339.

URAGUCHI, K. et al. 1961. Toxicological approach to the metabolites of Penicillium islandicum Sopp growing on the yellowed rice. Jpn. J. Exp. Med. 31, 1.

U.S. PUBLIC HEALTH SERV. 1974. Aflatoxins: Stopping trouble before it starts. U.S. Dep. Health, Educ. Welfare (FDA) 74–2050. U.S. Govt. Printing Off., Washington, D.C.

WILSON, B.J. and WILSON, C.H. 1962. Hepatotoxic substance from Penicillium rubrum. J. Bacteriol. 83, 693.

WOGAN, G.H. 1965. Mycotoxins in Food. M.I.T. Press, Cambridge, Mass.

20

Chemical Poisoning

Like the biologic contaminants (microbial, protozoan, and helminthic) of food and water, gastroenteritis of varying severity, often fatal, may be caused by the ingestion of toxic chemicals that may be present in food or drink. As the list of such chemicals is of great magnitude, our discussion will be limited to those that are most frequently encountered.

There are several ways in which these injurious chemicals may be ingested: (1) mistaken use of a toxic chemical in the preparation, seasoning, or sweetening of a food because of its close physical resemblance to a commonly used dietary product; (2) the use of utensils for the cooking or storage of food or drink from which soluble toxic chemicals may leach out; (3) the ingestion of fruits and vegetables with an excessive quantity of residual insecticide on their surface; (4) ingestion by children of accessible chemicals (aspirin, lye, bleach, cleaning fluids) believing them to be confectioneries or drinks; (5) the deliberate and malicious contamination of food or drink with a poisonous chemical by an unscrupulous person for some irrational reason; (6) the pollution of a water source with fertilizer, pesticide, herbicide, or defoliant while treating farmland or spraying fruit trees.

The incubation period of chemical poisoning is very short, ranging from several minutes to 1 hr. In most instances the triad of gastroenteritis—vomiting, abdominal cramps, and diarrhea—are the predominant symptoms. These disagreeable reactions serve a useful therapeutic purpose: the vomiting rids the stomach of the food or fluid with the irritating chemical, the cramps indicate that increased peristalsis is hurrying the toxic material along the intestinal tract, and the diarrhea evacuates it completely out of the digestive system. Thus, nature does the work of ipecac and purging.

CHEMICALS

Sodium Fluoride

Sodium fluoride, an insecticide used for eliminating cockroaches, is a chemical that has on occasion been mistaken for flour, sugar, baking soda, or salt and has been used in the preparation of food. Persons who ingested such food came down with the gastrointestinal triad, plus pallor, cold sweats, convulsions, and collapse, depending on the quantity of fluoride ingested.

Sodium Nitrite and Nitrate

The New York City Department of Health reported an outbreak involving 11 men who "salted" their breakfast food in a cafeteria using salt shakers containing a sodium nitrite that is used for the curing and preservation of meat. Cyanosis, a bluish discoloration of the skin due to deficient oxygenation of the blood, was the prominent symptom in addition to the enteritis. Nitrites are added in the processing of bacon and other meats. Infants whose formulae are prepared with water from wells contaminated with nitrites or nitrates from industrial or other sources similarly develop cyanosis (methemoglobinemia).

Metallic Poisoning

The cooking of acid foods such as apples, and the storage of sour drink (lemonade, orange juice) in certain types of pots, trays, or pitchers may result in metallic poisoning. If cheap gray cooking enamelware is used, antimony present in the enamel may leach out and cause poisoning giving rise to gastroenteritis. Acid foods cooked in copper pots may dissolve out a sufficient quantity of copper to cause vomiting. If cadmium-plated ice cube trays or pitchers are used with sour foods or drinks, such as orange juice, punch, or wine, the leached cadmium, when ingested, will cause illness. The zinc in galvanized ware may be dissolved by acid foods and give rise to the enteritis triad and pain in the mouth and throat.

Drinking water running through lead pipes, and acid foods injudiciously kept in lead vessels will leach out quantities of the metal and cause acute lead poisoning giving rise to abdominal and muscular cramps, vomiting, and diarrhea. In England, lead-lined vats for the brewing of beer caused a widespread outbreak of lead poisoning. If the ingestion of lead in food or drink is continued for some time, chronic lead poisoning with the characteristic blue line on the gums and wrist drop may result. Lead poisoning may be an occupational hazard to workers engaged in the production of paints, batteries, gasoline, pottery glazes, and insecticide sprays. Infants may poison themselves by gnawing the lead paint from window sills, their cribs, or toys.

Pesticides

For many years, man has conducted chemical warfare against the insects. The ammunition he has used against them in the preservation of one of his main sources of food has been the chemical insecticides which he has produced in many varieties. These chemicals are lethal to the insects and are also harmful to humans if accidentally ingested. Some of them, when fed to laboratory animals, have been found to be carcinogenic (capable of causing cancer) and others teratogenic (capable of producing abnormalities in the fetus). It therefore is important for us to exercise extreme caution in the handling and use of these toxic products. It is also necessary for us to remove thoroughly any residual of insecticide that may remain on the surface of fruits and vegetables that have been salvaged in the battle with these marauders.

Before the introduction of the chlorinated hydrocarbons and the organic phosphate insecticides, inorganic toxic elements, among them compounds such as arsenic, lead, mercury, barium, and fluorides, were employed. Some of them are still in use today. Apples, pears, and vegetables that have been sprayed with lead arsenate may still retain a residue when purchased. It is therefore necessary to wash these foods thoroughly before eating them.

The chlorinated hydrocarbons, among them DDT, DDE, DDD, chlordane, endrin, and toxophene, are effective insecticides, although it is now illegal to employ some of them. Residuals on leafy vegetables should be washed before ingestion. Food or utensils accidentally contaminated may cause headache, nausea, dizziness, confusion, and convulsions within half an hour after ingestion. Similarly, the organic phosphates such as DDP, DDVP, TEPP, diazinon, malathion, and parathion will also cause illness if any of them inadvertently contaminates food. Depending on the amount ingested, patients will complain within 5 min of headache, nausea, vomiting, diarrhea, salivation, blurred vision, cyanosis, nervousness, sweating, and chest and abdominal pains.

Barium carbonate, used as a rat poison, may be mistaken for flour and if the baked product is eaten, gastroenteritis with a tingling sensation of the face and neck, loss of tendon reflexes, muscular paralysis, and cardiac symptoms may result. Arsenic is also used as a rodenticide. The author (I.J.T.) investigated an outbreak of enteritis in 40 persons who had eaten coffee buns purchased at a local bakery. Arsenic was located in a sample of buns. Evidence was found that the poison had been introduced into an open sack of flour at the bakery by rats, as an exterminator had scattered several "rat balls" containing the poison along the floor on the previous afternoon.

Acute poisoning with bichloride of mercury, either by accidentally contaminated food or if taken deliberately with suicidal intent, may prove fatal within 2 to 30 min. Affected persons usually complain of an astringent metallic taste, burning pain in the mouth, excessive thirst, salivation, colicky pains, vomiting, and watery diarrhea.

Silver Polish

A number of silver polishes contain cyanide. If silver tableware is not sufficiently washed to remove residues of the polish, gastroenteritis with cold perspiration, cyanosis, mental confusion, and exhaustion may result when the silverware is used. Should an excessive quantity of polish contaminate the food that is ingested, death may result.

Nicotinic Acid

In order to restore the natural color to meats of inferior quality, unscrupulous dealers add nicotinic acid or sodium nitrate to it. The untoward action of nitrate has been described. Nicotinic acid applied in excessive quantity to meat will cause flushing of the face, neck, and upper extremities, a feeling of extreme heat, itching, headache, sweating, and occasionally nausea, vomiting, abdominal cramps, and diarrhea within 10 to 30 min following ingestion. Cooking the treated meat fails to destroy the action of the nicotinic acid.

Antibiotics

Attention is called to a growing risk to humans resulting from the use of antibiotics and certain hormones in the raising of farm animals. Although these chemicals cannot be considered to be poisonous, their extensive use in farm husbandry presents some problems. The reason that penicillin, tetracyclines, and other antibiotics given to some patients prove ineffective is due to their massive use in the feed of farm animals such as cattle, pigs, and chickens. These drugs protect the animals from disease and cause them to gain weight—a beneficial economical result. Antibiotics in animal feed have contributed to a growing pool of drug-resistant bacteria. As a result, physicians are finding a reduced effectiveness of the drugs in the treatment of disease. In 1971, the Food and Drug Administration (FDA) proposed a withdrawal of the routine use of penicillin and other antibiotics in animal feeds. Recently the Office of Technology Assessment, an arm of Congress, has reported that most of the drugs used in the feeds of farm animals could be replaced with alternate drugs already approved by the FDA.

Hormones

The use of DES (diethylstilbestrol), a synthetic female sex hormone, in order to promote growth in beef cattle is now banned by the FDA. The reason is that DES is a proven carcinogen capable of causing vaginal cancer in some of the daughters, as well as certain genital abnormalities in some of the sons, of women who received it during pregnancy. Although the Office of Technology Assessment stated that the amount of DES left in meat may not be sufficient to cause human cancer, there remain uncertainties in assessing the risk. From the humanitarian point of view, it would appear that the prevention of human illness and death is of greater importance than the production of increased quantities of meat.

Monosodium Glutamate

On April 4, 1968, a Chinese physician, Robert Ho Mau Kwok, on the staff of National Biomedical Research Foundation, Silver Spring, Maryland, wrote a letter to the editor of the New England Journal of Medicine in which he stated, "For several years since I have been in this country, I have experienced a strange syndrome whenever I have eaten out in a Chinese restaurant, especially one that served Northern Chinese food. The syndrome, which usually begins 15 to 20 minutes after I have eaten the first dish, lasts for about two hours, without any hangover effect. The most prominent symptoms are numbness at the back of the neck, gradually radiating to both arms and the back, general weakness and palpitations."

The letter apparently attracted sufficient attention among readers of the journal for a number of them to write to the editor describing similar symptoms in themselves and in members of their family or in patients upon ingestion of Chinese food. Various explanations were given for what was referred to as the Chinese Restaurant Syndrome. A number of items that go into the preparation of Chinese food were suspected: soy sauce, monosodium glutamate, cooking wine, Chinese vegetables, and high salt content.

A study conducted at the Albert Einstein College of Medicine revealed that monosodium glutamate was responsible for the syndrome, the larger the dose, the more intense the burning sensations, the facial pressure, and the chest pains. It was also found that some persons appeared more sensitive than others to the smaller doses.

As the prior ingestion of glutamate-free food will delay the absorption of the incriminated seasoning in the Chinese food, it is suggested that persons subject to the Chinese Restaurant Syndrome eat a few hors d'oeuvres shortly before going to their favorite Chinese restaurant.

The attention of the authors has been called to some unusual types of chemical poisonings. Among them was the occurrence of thallium poisoning of 4 residents who had eaten chicken soup at a lunchroom. It was found that an "ant-trap" kept on a shelf above the stove had fallen into the pot of soup. The chicken soup, considered by some to be a panacea, in this instance caused violent gastroenteritis. Diagnosis of thallium poisoning was suspected when it was noted that all 4 patients developed alopecia (loss of hair), and it was later confirmed by laboratory tests.

An investigation was also made of a report by a school physician that a number of high school students had complained of a burning sensation of the lips and mouth upon biting into pretzels that each had purchased. On inspection of the bakery, it was learned that the raw pretzels pass through a weak solution of lye before baking in order to produce their attractive glossy brown coloring. Too much lye had apparently been used in the preparation of that batch of pretzels.

Prevention

The accidental ingestion of toxic chemicals may be prevented by exercising care in their storage and use. Household and garden chemicals should be stored separately from food products and should be kept out of the reach of young children. Manufacturers who put up their toxic (as well as medicinal) products in containers with tops or caps that cannot be opened by children (and even by some adults!) are rendering a commendable service to the public health. The use of colored dyes in toxic products, such as the insecticides, would greatly minimize their being mistaken for useful nutritive items. Because of the toxicity of the insecticides to humans, studies are being conducted to find less hazardous means for the control of destructive insects. Thought is being given to Integrated Pest Management (IPM) in which use is made of such measures as the dissemination of predatory insects to feed on the undesirable ones, the use of bacteria and viruses that are lethal to crop-destroying insects but harmless to man, and the production of insect-resistant crops.

The use of kitchen utensils, pots, trays, and containers of questionable quality should be avoided. Stainless steel ware, although more expensive, is the most desirable and safest ware.

All fruits that are not peelable and all leafy vegetables should be thoroughly washed before they are eaten in order to remove all residual insecticide on their surface.

Treatment

Detailed information regarding the treatment of chemical poisoning may be obtained in any standard textbook on toxicology. Briefly, the treatment involves the following general principles and procedures:

(1) Evacuation of the bulk of the ingested poison as promptly as possible from the stomach and intestinal tract by gastric lavage, emetics (mustard in water, suds of laundry soap, syrup of ipecac), or cathartics (magnesium sulphate). However, it is not always advisable to pass a stomach tube for gastric lavage or to induce vomiting, as some corrosive chemicals (such as lye) may severely damage the esophagus and stomach which may be further damaged during lavage or vomiting.

(2) Use of specific antidotes orally by stomach tube or parenterally (intravenously or subcutaneously).

(3) Elimination of poison already absorbed by forcing fluids orally or parenterally.

(4) Symptomatic treatment.

(5) In some instances it may be necessary to make use of hemodialysis (artificial kidney).

Information on household and industrial chemicals may be obtained through poison control centers in all parts of the United States. For the location of the nearest center call your local department of health.

Prison Outbreak of Gastroenteritis

Three outbreaks of acute gastroenteritis involving a total of approximately 1600 inmates of a prison are mentioned because of their unusual causative factor and method of transmission. The chemical and epidemiologic patterns in all three were remarkably similar, even to the extent of developing at the same time of day on the same day of the week on each occasion.

On epidemiologic investigation made by members of the New York State Department of Health, it was found that illness was limited to men who had consumed 1 or more of 4 different foods served at 2 different meals. Meat stock prepared in one large kettle and poured over meat slices that had been heated, also made into gravy for potatoes, as well as used in soup was common to the 4 foods. The soup and gravy proved toxic when fed to mice and had pH values above 13. Commercial caustic soda issued to plumbers from one of the prison industries for cleaning plugged floor drains could have been introduced into the meat stock as a malicious act. It was not known whether the irritant effect on the gastrointestinal mucosa was due to the alkalinity, to the impurities in the crude commercial caustic soda, or to compounds formed by the alkaline reaction with the foods.

Treatment in the Home

Studies have shown that chemical poisoning is one of the major causes of mortality and morbidity in children under 5 years of age with most of the poisoning involving the ingestion of household products or non-prescription drugs.

It is therefore important that parents be informed regarding poison prevention and how to deal effectively with intoxication in a child. They should be aware of certain signs and symptoms that may indicate poisoning and should know what initial steps must be taken. They should suspect poisoning if they note unusual sleepiness, strange behavior, unusual odors, and seizures in a non-epileptic or afebrile child. They should look for spilled medication or household agent or other evidence of toxic ingestion.

If the child is fully awake, a dose of syrup of ipecac to induce vomiting, and copious fluids may be given. The most available antidote is milk, as in large quantities it will help neutralize corrosive effects, delay gastric emptying to the intestine, and act as a diluent.

A phone call to the Poison Control Center, if the family physician is not immediately available, will bring information regarding what treatment should be given promptly. The physician may then institute appropriate therapy, such as proper technique of gastric emptying, use of the recommended antidote, and general supportive treatment.

Mother's Milk

Breast-feeding of infants, although recommended by physicians for its advantages over formula infant feeding, may also prove hazardous to the infant should the mother be taking certain drugs during the period of time that she is nursing her baby. A number of prescription and over-the-counter drugs pass into the breast milk and may prove toxic to the nursing infant. This is especially true of drugs with inherent toxicity in themselves, such as antineoplastic agents, radioactive compounds, and the heavy metals.

A study conducted at the Poison Center of the Nassau County Medical Center by Mofenson and Greensher (1980), and supported by a grant from the National Foundation-March of Dimes, revealed that a significant number of drugs taken by the mother, even in usual doses, carry a potential or a considerable risk to the nursing infant and that such drugs should be avoided by the nursing mother.

A report of the study appeared in the Winter 1980 issue of NCMC Proceedings, a quarterly publication of the Nassau County Medical Center. It lists over 50 drugs that fall into that category. Among them are the antibiotics streptomycin, tetracyclines, chloramphenicol, and novobiocin; the anticoagulant phenindione; the antithyroid drugs thiouracil and iodides; the antihypertensive drugs reserpine and propranolol; the antirheumatic drugs indomethacin, butazones, and aspirin in large doses; the cardiac medicines atropine and quinine; the central nervous system stimulant nicotine (20 to 30 cigarettes per day); the depressants heroin, alcohol, chloral hydrate, and bromides; and the tranquilizers chlorpromazine, diazepam, meprobamate, and lithium. The chronic use of large doses of corticosteroids should be avoided. Sulfonamides should be taken by the mother only after the infant is over 2 months of age. Even laxatives such as cascara, rhubarb, and aloes if taken by the mother may cause loose stools in the infant.

FOOD ADDITIVES

The U.S. Food, Drug and Cosmetic Act defines a food additive as a substance the intended use of which results, or may be reasonably expected to result, directly or indirectly, in its becoming a component or otherwise affecting the characteristics of any food. They are intentionally added to food, generally in small quantities, to improve their appearance, flavor, texture, and storage properties. The Food and Drug Administration (FDA) lists 31 categories of food additives, among them colorings, antioxidants, acidulants, flavor enhancers, emulsifiers, enzymes, leavening agents, antispoilants, thickeners, supplemental preservatives, agents to delay or enhance the ripening of fruits and vegetables, agents to increase or decrease moisture in foods, nutrition supplements (vitamins, minerals, amino acids), and artificial sweeteners. They are used to provide essential aids in food processing, make food more attractive to the consumer, maintain and improve the nutritional quality of food, and, by enhancing its keeping quality, reduce the waste of food.

There are more than 2000 chemicals used as direct additives to food. It is estimated that more than 363 million kg (800 million lb) of such chemicals are added to processed foods each year, with each person in the United States consuming between 1.8 and 2.3 kg (4 and 5 lb) of the additives in such foods as TV dinners, snack foods, and frozen foods.

The law requires that food and chemical manufacturers run extensive animal feeding tests on all additives before they are marketed, and FDA scientists must be satisfied that the additive in question is not harmful. It is then designated as "generally recognized as safe" (GRAS). Some of these chemicals in food may not cause immediate acute illness, but it may take several years, or even a lifetime of exposure to learn their long-term effect on consumers. Some may prove in time to be carcinogenic or mutagenic or teratogenic.

The Food Additive Amendment, Public Health Law *85-929*, introduced by Congressman James Delaney and passed in 1958, specifies that no additive may be permitted in any amount in food if tests show that it produces cancer when fed to man or animals or by any other appropriate test (U.S. Food Drug Admin. 1958).

A number of additives on the GRAS list that were subsequently found to be carcinogenic to laboratory animals were banned after they had been used for varying periods of time. Among them are a number of food dyes previously approved as "U.S. Certified Colors"; the artificial sweeteners cyclamate and dulcin; the synthetic hormone diethylstilbestrol (DES) that had been added to animal feed to promote growth and used to caponize poultry; the flavorings, oil of calamus and safrol (from sassafras bark used in root beer); and diethylpyrocarbonate (DEP), used as a preservative in many carbonated drinks. The ingestion of nitrites present in cured meats acts as a deterrent to the growth of *C. botulinum* in the meat. However, the nitrite may interact with secondary and tertiary amines and amides in the body and form nitrosamines that are believed to be carcinogenic.

Other previously approved chemicals that have been found to be toxic to humans have also been banned. Cobalt salts, used as a stabilizer and antigushing agent in beer, have been found to cause fatal heart attacks. Coumarin, an artificial flavoring in synthetic vanilla extract, was found to cause liver damage in rats and dogs after it had been in use for many years. Lithium chloride, a salt substitute, was banned after causing several fatalities. An antibrowning agent used with frozen sliced fruit proved toxic and was also banned.

As in the case of foods that naturally contain small amounts of toxic chemicals, as described in Chapter 22, most of the additives in processed foods also appear in such minimal quantities that acute poisoning seldom occurs. However, possible adverse effects may result if the ingested quantity of chemical is increased by appearing in foods consumed in subtantial amounts each day, such as bread, milk, meat, and fruit, rather than in foods eaten only occasionally and in small amounts. Nonetheless, allergists point out that no matter how small the quantity of additive may be, with some individuals each new compound that is ingested may prove to be a potential invitation to an allergic or anaphylactic reaction.

Food processors claim that by adding chemicals to food they are able to maintain or improve nutritional quality, make certain foods more attractive, retard decay and spoilage, and reduce waste by lengthening their keeping and storage time. Additives, however, should not be used to deceive the consumer by disguising faulty processing and handling, or to replace good manufacturing practices which could accomplish the same effect.

Food processors and manufacturers maintain that foods containing low levels of additives are safe. This is questioned by a number of authorities, among them Franklin Bicknell, M.D. (1960), who suggests that there may be a cause-and-effect relationship between food additives and the incidence of the degenerative diseases. He has stated:

Americans consume more chemicals in their food than any other nation. At the same time American forecasts are the gloomiest in the world about the continued rise of cancer, high blood pressure, heart disease, congenital abnormalities, etc.: in fact, all the degenerative diseases. The United States leads the civilized world in chemicalized food and in degenerative diseases.

Public health personnel involved in the investigation of chemical food poisoning may find it helpful to observe how the following two investigations were conducted.

INVESTIGATION OF ARSENICAL POISONING AT DRIVE-IN THEATER IN MASSAPEQUA, N.Y., ON AUGUST 21, 1954

Reason for Investigation

On Saturday, August 21, at 12:30 P.M., Dr. G.C.E., Assistant Superintendent, Meadowbrook Hospital, East Meadow, N.Y., telephoned the senior author at his home and reported that at 1:45 A.M. that morning 7 cases of severe gastroenteritis had been admitted to the hospital. All had become ill at the drive-in theater at Massapequa, N.Y. Five were employed at the theater and 2 were patrons.

Investigation

The author promptly visited the hospital and found the patients to be as follows:

	Name	Address	Age	Occupation
(1)	T.G.	Massapequa Park, N.Y.	29	Counterman
(2)	J.R.	Queens Village, N.Y.	50	Concession Manager
(3)	J.B.	Seaford, N.Y.	27	Concession Worker

	Name	Address	Age	Occupation
(4)	R.M.	No. Merrick, N.Y.	19	Asst. Pro-jectionist
(5)	F.B.	Massapequa Park, N.Y.	27	Concession Worker
(6)	R.S.	Brooklyn, N.Y.	17	Patron
(7)	R.W.	Woodhaven, N.Y.	19	Patron

Each patient stated that he had had 1 or more drinks of cola at the movie concession. No other article of food or drink was taken in common by them, 6 having had dinner at their respective homes and 1 at a cafeteria before arriving at the theater.

The author visited the drive-in theater at about 3 P.M. It was learned that approximately 200 cola drinks had been sold the evening of August 20 during the half-hour intermission between 10:00 and 10:30 P.M. During that time many patrons left their cars and went to the concession in order to purchase any of the following items: cola drinks, orange drinks, frankfurters, hamburgers, Chinese shrimp egg-rolls, popcorn, packaged candy bars, ice cream dixie cups, and ice cream sandwiches. Cola is served from 3 dispensing fountains, one being located at each end and one in the center of the counter. During the intermission, the employees were busy serving the patrons and at its termination they cleaned up as usual and refilled the vats of each of the dispensers with cola syrup in preparation for the following evening. The syrup is purchased in 0.95 liter (1 gal.) bottles, 4 per carton.

Clinical Character of Illness

Illness was characterized by sudden onset of nausea and severe repeated vomiting and retching, gastralgia, colic, and prostration. Two patients on admission to the hospital were in severe shock and had to be given intravenous infusion of plasma. Cyanosis was noted in 3 patients and 1 had diarrhea. Four patients complained of burning sensation of the throat. Gastric lavage was performed promptly on admission and all received intravenous infusions of saline and glucose solutions.

Incubation Period

Although one of the patients (T.G.) had 2 cola drinks before the intermission, all 7 patients, including T.G., had a drink after the intermission. At about 11:00 P.M., R.M., the assistant projectionist, and J.B., concession worker, each drank a cola. About 10 to 15 min later, their throats became sore; they felt nauseated and went to the men's toilet where they vomited violently. At 11:15 P.M. 2 patrons, R.S. and R.W., purchased cola drinks but after taking several sips they complained about the taste and a burning sensation of the throat. They returned the drinks and received orange drinks in exchange. About 10 min later they also had nausea, severe vomiting, and abdominal cramps.

When the attention of the manager, J.R., was called to these attacks, he and two other employees, F.B. and T.G., decided to sample the drinks from the left and center dispensers. They agreed that the drinks drawn from the former had a bad taste ("like carbolic acid") and J.R. ordered the syrup in that vat poured down the sink drain. Within 10 to 15 min the 3 tasters became ill.

Additional Cases

As the illness of the 7 patients was becoming more severe, they were transported by automobile to Meadowbrook Hospital where treatment for acute poisoning was promptly administered. The theater manager, H.C., drew a sample from the suspected fountain and took it to the hospital for analysis. The sample was diluted and amber colored, as the syrup in the vat of that fountain had been emptied and the drink contained only the small quantity of syrup which remained in the mixing valve and in the line which is about 20 cm (8 in.) long. H.C. also tasted the drink, taking only one sip. He vomited several times about 3 hr later.

The manager of the theater that night contacted the representative of the cola company who resides in Hicksville, N.Y. He arrived at the theater at 3 A.M. promptly and emphatically exonerated his product, and to prove the confidence he had in the preparation he sold, drew himself a drink from the middle fountain and drank "about one table-spoon" of it. He admitted that the drink did have a "metallic taste— probably due to the action of the carbonic acid on the lining of the metal tubing." He removed a number of empty syrup bottles to be sent to the laboratory of the cola company for analysis of the small quantity of syrup they contained. About 7 hr later (at 10:30 A.M.), the cola representative had cramps and vomited 6 times.

It was learned subsequently that 2 more employees of the theater, H.F. residing in Massapequa and M.S. from Amityville, had reported for treatment for vomiting and abdominal cramps to the emergency ward of the Meadowbrook Hospital on the afternoon of August 21. In addition, an unidentified patron was reported to have vomited several times in the men's room at about the time the other cases occurred. This makes a total of 12 persons known to have been made ill.

A telephone call to the police precinct in that area failed to reveal additional cases. The fire department emergency ambulance in Massapequa had not been summoned that day to transport any case to the hospital.

Causative Agent

As the cola drink was the only item of food or drink which all 11 persons involved in this outbreak from whom a history was obtained had in common, it appears that cola was most probably responsible for the outbreak. No illness was reported among the approximately 200 patrons who had cola drinks before the intermission. It may therefore be assumed that the causative agent was not present in the dispensing machine or machines at that time but was probably introduced after the intermission.

In view of the short "incubation period" (10 to 20 min in 7 patients), with sudden onset of severe vomiting and abdominal cramps as the prominent symptoms, the possibility of a chemical poison as the causative agent strongly suggested itself.

Control Measures

The dispensing machines were ordered disconnected and the carbon dioxide cylinders and the supply of cola syrup bottles embargoed. The acting concession manager was instructed not to dispense any fountain drinks (neither cola nor orange drinks) except such as come in bottles, cans, or containers.

Since the water supply is from a private well, its use for drinking purposes was prohibited until after samples had been analyzed and found to be potable.

As an incidental occurrence, it was found that apparently during the excitement of the outbreak, a refrigerator containing about 800 Chinese shrimp egg rolls had been disconnected the night before and had remained so for over 12 hr. Its temperature was found to be 17.8°C (64°F) and the shrimp rolls were embargoed and denatured following dumping into the garbage truck.

Laboratory Examinations

A portion of the diluted cola drink brought to Meadowbrook Hospital was obtained for examination at the Division of Laboratories & Research, Nassau County Department of Health. Arsenic in large quantity was reported by both the toxicological laboratory at the hospital and the Health Department Laboratory.

A thorough search for additional evidence and samples was made on the premises of the theater on August 23 and 24. With the aid of the representative of the distributor of the dispensing machines, additional samples were collected and examined at the Department of Health Laboratory with the following results:

Lab. No.	Material	Date Collected	Pertinent Information	Result of Examination
7111	Cola syrup	8-24-54	Sealed bottle—Lot #4K160805	Arsenic not detected
7112	Cola syrup	8-24-54	Sealed bottle—Lot #4K150805	Arsenic not detected
7114	Cola drainage		This material was the overflow collected from drain of center machine. This machine was presumably used by one of the cases.	Arsenic was detected in large quantities
7115	Cola drink		Sample #1—Another sample from valve of machine located on left end of counter facing from rear. Sample collected by company representative.	Arsenic detected in large quantities
7116	Cola drink		Sample #2—(Cola syrup + carbonated water) collected from left machine. This sample was collected 8-22-54.	Arsenic detected in large quantities
7117	Carbonated water		Sample #3—Carbonated water (containing no syrup)[1] was collected by company representative from machine located on left end.	Arsenic detected in large quantities
7118	Cola drink		Sample #4—Mixed drink collected by company representative from same left machine after machine had been checked and cleaned.	Arsenic detected in large quantities

[1] As the carbonated water passed through the mixing valve in which some residue of syrup might have been present, it cannot be considered to be straight carbonated water.

Lab. No.	Material	Date Collected	Pertinent Information	Result of Examination
7119	Cola syrup[2]		Composite sample from center and right end machines[2] before machines were emptied and cleaned, and after illness was reported. Sample was collected by company representative.	Arsenic detected in large quantities

Repeated examinations of the tap water at the theater failed to reveal the presence of arsenic.

Source of Arsenic

An attempt was made to determine how the arsenic got into the cola drinks. No insecticide or other poison with the exception of a partially-filled spray gun for fly spraying was found. The manager stated it had not been used for several months and denied that any work by a professional exterminator had been done for at least 3 months. A further search, however, revealed one partially filled [about 37.85 liters (10 gal.)] and one nearly empty 208 liter (55 gal.) metal drum of Dolge SS Weed Killer in the rear of the building. The latter had some rainwater in it since the tap holes were open. Samples were taken from each of these drums and examined at the Department of Health laboratory. *Arsenic was found in "high concentration"* in the weed killer, and "in very heavy quantities" in the diluted sample. The formula of the weed killer was obtained from the C.B. Dolge Company of Westport, Conn., its manufacturer. It contained sodium arsenite 38.0%; total arsenic expressed as metallic all water soluble 24.5%; inert ingredients—water 62.0%.

It was learned from the assistant theater manager that on August 18, 3 days before the outbreak, a 0.95 liter (1 gal.) bottle of cola syrup had been found near the movie screen by some children playing in that area. They notified a rampman who located it and took it to the concession where it was locked up in the desk. On the following day, August 19, it was turned over to the concession manager who placed it on top of the refrigerator where it remained until August 20. At about 8:00 P.M. it was moved to the back room and later placed on the top of a refrigerated chest behind the counter. T.G., who refilled the dispensing syrup vats after the intermission that evening at 10:30 P.M., definitely recalled using that bottle plus 2 others which he removed from a carton. He

---

[2] It is regrettable that separate samples of syrup from each machine had not been obtained.

emptied the contents of the retrieved 0.95 liter (1 gal.) bottle into the vats of the left and center dispensers. Neither he nor the manager remembers whether or not the seal of that bottle was broken.

Sabotage

The question of intentional poisoning of the cola drinks was given consideration. One cannot help agreeing with the representative of the cola company that had the adulterant been present in the syrup when it had left the manufacturer, similar outbreaks would have occurred in many other places where syrup from the same lot was sold. Direct adulteration at the movie concession could have been made only by one of the employees as they alone had access to the stockroom and the dispensing machines. It was learned that the relationship of the present employees of the theater and the concession with the management and each other had been most amicable. One employee, however, who was suspected of pilfering from the concession and who boasted on occasion of being able to pick locks, had been discharged about 3 weeks previous to the outbreak.

In view of the high concentration of arsenic reported in the drinks, it was feared that possible fatal poisoning had occurred and escaped detection. The county medical examiner was alerted to consider the possibility of arsenic poisoning in deaths which came to his attention within the next week or so.

The writer also conferred on August 25th with the assistant district attorney and police inspector, and the possible criminal aspect of the situation was discussed. Two detectives were assigned to investigate and question any suspects.

Conclusion

Eleven persons and one unidentified man came down with arsenic poisoning after having cola drinks dispensed at the drive-in theater in Massapequa, New York, on August 21, 1954. As these persons became ill after the 10:00 P.M. intermission, it is evident that the poison was introduced into the dispensers after that time. The adulteration must have occurred when syrup was added to the vats of the dispensing machines at about 10:30 P.M. The contents of a 0.95 liter (1 gal.) bottle of cola syrup found on the theater grounds 2 days before had been used to refill 2 of the machines. As none of the individuals who handled that bottle noted whether or not the seal was broken, it is probable that it contained the arsenic. The source of the arsenic is believed to be weed killer, a quantity of which was found on the premises.

It is probable that someone for some reason, perhaps to do damage to the business of the drive-in theater or to avenge himself upon the concession owner, introduced weed killer into a pilfered 0.95 liter (1 gal.) bottle of cola syrup. He then concealed it on the theater grounds with the intention of later replacing it in the storeroom or with the hope that it would be found, as actually occurred, and returned to the concession. Probably the culprit did not know that the weed killer contained as deadly a poison as arsenic. He might have intended merely to spoil the taste of the drinks and thus cause the mischief that he sought.

It is fortunate that the adulterated bottle of syrup had not been emptied into the dispensing machines before the intermission during which approximately 200 persons purchased cola drinks.

THE CASE OF THE 11 VOMITING CADDIES

On April 3rd, at 3:40 P.M., the manager of a country club located in Manhasset, New York, anxiously telephoned the Nassau County Department of Health and reported that 11 caddies employed at the golf course had suddenly become ill with severe abdominal cramps and vomiting. He had notified the club physician who had recommended that the health authorities be promptly informed. An investigation was immediately started in order to determine the cause of the outbreak and to take steps to prevent the occurrence of additional cases.

Probable Cause of Illness

It was found that illness was characterized by sudden onset of nausea and severe vomiting, retching, and marked abdominal cramps. One of the caddies' vomitus was blood-tinged. Early that afternoon, each patient had had a carbonated drink from a coin-operated vending machine located in the caddies' locker room. The machine dispensed 4 different beverages in individual paper cups: cola, root beer, orange drink, and grape drink. The drinks were available with or without crushed ice. The machine was plugged into an electric outlet and a copper tube from the machine was connected to a water pipe.

One of the caddies had purchased a drink of root beer without ice at 10:30 A.M. with no ill effect. He bought a similar drink at 12:30 P.M. and this was followed by severe vomiting 15 min later. Another caddy had a cola drink with no ice at noon without any effect. A similar drink at 1 P.M. induced abdominal cramps and vomiting within 10 min. The remaining 9 caddies had various flavored drinks, some with and others without ice, in the early afternoon. All became ill within 10 to 15 min.

The caddies with 2 exceptions resided in different parts of Nassau County and New York City. They had not eaten the same breakfast or lunch or any other food in common that day, but all had had one or more drinks from the vending machine. It therefore appeared highly probable that their illness was caused by the drinks dispensed by the machine. The brief incubation period between the drinking and the onset of illness strongly suggested that a chemical poison was most probably responsible for the acute gastroenteritis.

Vending Machine

An embargo tag was placed on the dispensing machine. Its owner was contacted by telephone and requested to send someone to the club promptly to open the machine for inspection so that samples of the different syrups, ice, and carbonated water could be obtained for laboratory examination.

The machine produced its own ice and carbonated the water with compressed carbon dioxide from a tank. It was observed that the ice as well as the carbonated water had a bright yellow-orange color. The valve on the line of the water entering the machine was opened and a sample of water was obtained before it was frozen or carbonated. It also had the orange coloring. The copper pipe which conveyed the water to the machines was thereupon followed. On touching it, it felt warm as if it contained hot water. It ran through the wall into the boiler room where it was connected to one of a number of pipes running along the ceiling. A valve at the connection was opened and a sample of water taken. It proved to be hot and had the same orange color as the samples taken from the machine. For comparison, samples of both hot and cold water were taken from the faucets of the wash basins in the caddies' toilet room adjacent to their locker room, as well as from the salad sink in the club's kitchen. These appeared colorless, as potable water should be.

Improper Water Connection

On questioning the club maintenance man, it was learned that the copper pipe which supplied the water to the vending machine was not connected to a pipe in which potable water ran but had been joined to the hot water recirculating line which is part of the hot water heating system and runs to the radiators in the club building. He stated that he had not been aware of this connection and had not been consulted at the time it was made. He then revealed a crucial piece of information. He said that on the previous day, April 2nd, between 4 and 5 P.M., he had added 2 gal. of a corrosion and rust-preventing chemical to the recirculating hot water system. The label on the metal drum containing the preparation indicated that it was called Kem Kool and that it was produced by the

Chem Testing Corporation located in Queens, New York City. An unsuccessful attempt was made to reach the producer by telephone on the evening of the investigation.

Causative Agent

A telephone call was then made to the Poison Control Center at Meadowbrook Hospital, East Meadow, N.Y., in order to determine the nature of the toxic chemicals in Kem Kool. The center had no information regarding the composition of Kem Kool but it stated that most rust preventives usually contain dichromate. The universal antidote of drinking milk and inducing vomiting was recommended. This information was promptly relayed to the physician at the club. Subsequent information obtained from the producer revealed that each 56.8 liter (15 gal.) drum of Kem Kool contained 22.7 kg (50 lb) of sodium dichromate, 2.3 kg (5 lb) of trisodium phosphate, and 11.4 liters (3 gal.) of 50% solution of sodium hydroxide. Two gal. (7.6 liters) of Kem Kool added to the 1893 or 2271 liters (500 or 600 gal.) of water in the recirculating hot water system resulted in a concentration of 440 ppm of hexavalent chromium as was subsequently determined by the Division of Laboratories and Research, Nassau County Department of Health. The hydrogen ion concentration (pH) was found to be 12.39. The carbonated water contained 420 ppm of hexavalent chromium and had a pH of 6.28, the difference being due to the chemical reaction with carbonic acid and the neutralization of the sodium hydroxide in the Kem Kool. Analysis of the samples of cold and hot water taken from the tap of the wash basin in the caddies' room and from the club kitchen revealed them to be within normal limits, containing less than 0.01 ppm of hexavalent chromium and the pH being within neutral limits (Table 20.1).

TABLE 20.1. LABORATORY ANALYSIS OF WATER SAMPLES

Source of Water	Hexavalent Chromium (ppm)	pH
Vending machine (plain water)	440.0	12.39
Vending machine (carbonated water)	420.0	6.28
Wash basin, caddies' room (cold water)	<0.01	6.16
Wash basin, caddies' room (hot water)	<0.01	6.53
Kitchen salad sink (hot and cold water)	<0.01	6.46

It is interesting to note that the first 2 caddies to purchase drinks early that day were not made ill at that time although the anti-rust solution had been added to the recirculating water system about 18 hr before. They did become ill, however, when they drank from the machine sometime later. Apparently the water in their first drink was the residual in the copper water inlet pipe and within the machine. The toxic chemical solution had not yet reached the dispensing portion of the machine.

Amateur Plumbing

The vending machine had been installed in the caddies' locker room approximately 1 year before the occurrence of the outbreak. The connection to the source of water supply was made by an employee of the vending corporation who is not only unlicensed for the making of permanent plumbing connections, but is not even a plumber. Apparently he had neither consulted the plans of the plumbing layout of the club in order to determine which pipe contained potable water nor had he solicited such information from the club maintenance man. As a result, patrons purchasing drinks from the machine had been drinking, for a period of 1 year, water from a recirculating hot water system which was carbonated, flavored with syrup, and cooled with cracked ice. The addition of the rust-preventive solution to the heating system revealed this fact grievously.

Control Measures

The representative of the vending corporation was promptly ordered to shut off the dispensing mechanism in the machine, to disconnect the copper water inlet tube from the recirculating hot water system, and to remove the machine as soon as practicable. It was recommended that the pipes, coils, and tanks within the machine be thoroughly cleaned and flushed before it was put back in operation. When it was reinstalled, it was to be properly connected to a cold potable water pipe by a licensed plumber. The Health Department sanitarian has subsequently ascertained that these instructions have been carried out.

Progress Note

Although a number of the caddies who drank from the machine were severely ill, it is fortunate that the spontaneous vomiting was so prompt and intense that apparently little, if any, of the toxic chemicals remained in their stomachs as evidenced by their rapid recovery. Eight of the caddies returned to work on the following day. The club physician stated that as far as he knew, the other 3 caddies also recovered with no ill effect.

Discussion

This outbreak illustrates the necessity of more intense supervision of the installation, servicing, and operation of food and drink vending coin machines. Such machines dispensing a variety of hot and cold foods and drinks are extremely popular and are constantly being placed in large numbers in public places. Their faulty installation, as described in this book, or their improper operation may prove a health hazard.

The tapping of the water inlet of a drink-dispensing machine into a water supply should be made by a competent artisan. Once installed, frequent inspections and periodic servicing should be made to maintain the machine in a sanitary condition and to make certain that it functions properly.

There is another avoidable hazard, namely, copper poisoning, which may occur if drinks are consumed from a malfunctioning dispensing machine. Carbonated soft drink vending machines have a double check valve which prevents carbon dioxide from backing up into the main water system. Should the valve be defective—become obstructed or held open by foreign matter—carbon dioxide gas would be vented into the copper tubing connecting the machine with the water supply. When such backflow occurs, a chemical reaction takes place between the gas and the tubing, introducing into the drink soluble copper carbonate, which may prove toxic in excessive concentration.

What may be needed is more rigid control, such as the adoption of an ordinance or code which would provide for the licensing of vending machine operations. This would establish better liaison between the health officer and the machine operators and would result in more meaningful inspections and circumvent some of the unfortunate sanitation and safety problems that have occurred in the past.

Summary

A vending machine dispensing drinks, in operation for about a year at a country club, was improperly connected to the recirculating hot water heating system. Anti-rust solution containing sodium dichromate, trisodium phosphate, and sodium hydroxide added to the heating system was dispensed in the drinks causing acute gastroenteritis in 11 persons who purchased drinks from the machine. All recovered with no fatality.

REFERENCES

ANON. 1974. Drugs in breast milk. Med. Lett. *16* (25).

ANON. 1978. The risk/benefit concept as applied to food. Food Technol. *32* (3) 51.

AYERS, J.C., KRAFT, A.A., SNYDER, H.E. and WALKER, H.W. 1962. Chemical and Biologic Hazards in Food. Iowa State Univ. Press, Ames.

BANWART, G.J. 1979. Basic Food Microbiology. AVI Publishing Co., Westport, Conn.

BICKNELL, F. 1960. Chemicals in Food and Farm Products: Their Harmful Effects. Faber and Faber, London. (see American edition)

BINKERD, E.F. and KOLARI, O.E. 1975. The history and use of nitrate and nitrite in the curing of meat. Food Cosmet. Toxicol. *13*, 655.

COMMUNICABLE DIS. CENT. 1975. Acute nitrite poisoning. Morbidity Mortality *24*, 195.

DACK, G.M. 1956. Food Poisoning, 3rd Edition. Univ. of Chicago Press, Chicago.

DESROSIER, N.W. and DESROSIER, J.N. 1977. The Technology of Food Preservation, 4th Edition. AVI Publishing Co., Westport, Conn.

FASSETT, D.W. 1966. Nitrates and nitrites. *In* Toxicants Occurring Naturally in Foods. Natl. Acad. Sci./Natl. Res. Counc. Publ. *1354*.

GOSSELIN, R.E., HODGE, H.C., SMITH, R.P. and GLEASON, M.W. 1976. Clinical Toxicology of Commercial Products: Acute Poisoning, 4th Edition. Williams & Wilkins Co., Baltimore.

HUNTER, B.T. 1975. The Mirage of Safety. Charles Scribner's Sons, New York.

KELLER, E.L. 1979. Poisoning in children. Postgrad. Med. *25*, 177.

KINGSBURY, J.M. 1964. Poisonous Plants of the United States and Canada. Prentice-Hall, Englewood Cliffs, N.J.

MAXEY, J.O. and ROSENAU, J.J. 1965. Preventive Medicine and Public Health. P.E. Sartwell (Editor). Appleton-Century-Crofts, New York.

MERCK AND CO. 1977. The Merck Manual of Diagnosis and Therapy, 13th Edition. Merck, Sharp and Dohme Research Laboratories, Division of Merck and Co., Rahway, N.J.

MIDDLEKAUF, R.D. 1974. Legalities concerning food additives. Food Technol. *28* (5) 42.

MOFENSON, H.C. and GREENSHER, J. 1980. Mother's medication. A hazard to nursing infant. Nassau County Med. Cent. Proc. 7 (1) 1.

NATL. RES. COUNC. 1973. Toxicants Occurring Naturally in Foods, 2nd Edition. National Academy of Sciences, Washington, D.C.

ORGERON, D. *et al.* 1959. Methemoglobinemia from eating meat with high nitrite content. Public Health Rep. *72*, 189.

PERIGO, J.A. and ROBERTS, T.A. 1968. Inhibition of clostridia by nitrite. J. Food Technol. *3*, 91.

SCHAUMBURG, H.H., BYCK, R., GERSTL, R. and MASHMAN, J.H. 1969. Monosodium glutamate: Its pharmacology and role in the Chinese restaurant syndrome. Science *163*, 826.

SEN, N.P. *et al.* 1974. Effect of additives on the formation of nitrosamines in meat curing mixture containing spices and nitrites. J. Agric. Food Chem. *22*, 1125.

SPIHER, A.T., JR. 1971. The GRAS List Review. Reprint from Food Drug Admin. Pap., Dec. 1970–Jan. 1971.

TARTAKOW, I.J. 1969. Eleven vomiting caddies. Am. J. Public Health *59*, 1674.

TARTAKOW, I.J. 1977. Casebook of a medical detective: A review of interesting cases. Nassau County Med. Cent. *4* (2) 65–73.

TETRAULT, R.C. and PETTET, C.B. 1962. Chemical Food Poisoning California. Natl. Communicable Dis. Cent., Atlanta. Morbidity Mortality Weekly Rep. *23*, 178.

THIENES, C.R. and HALEY, T.J. 1972. Clinical Toxicology, 5th Edition. Lea and Febiger, Philadelphia.

U.S. DEP. HEALTH, EDUC. WELFARE, PUBLIC HEALTH SERV. 1963. Clinical Handbook on Economic Poisons. National Communicable Disease Center, Atlanta.

U.S. FOOD DRUG ADMIN. 1958. Food Additive Amendment to Federal Food, Drug and Cosmetic Act of 1938. ("Delaney Clause.") Public Health Law *85-929*. Sept. 6.

VISEK, W.J., CLINTON, S.K. and TRUEX, O.R. 1978. Nutrition and experimental carcinogenesis. Cornell Vet. *68*, 3.

WALTON, G. 1951. Survey of literature relating to infants with methemoglobinemia due to nitrate contaminated water. Am. J. Public Health *41*, 986.

WINTER, R. 1971. Beware of the Food You Eat. Crown Publishers, New York.

WRIGHT, H.N. 1963. An Outline of Toxicology. Univ. Bookstores, Univ. of Minnesota, Minneapolis.

21

Poisonous Plants

Plants, especially those in the flower garden, are beautiful to behold, and are considered by most of us to be innocuous. However, a number of them have been found to be poisonous if certain of their parts are ingested. The U.S. Public Health Service reports that about 12,000 children are made ill each year by eating potentially poisonous plants.

Poisonous plants are present everywhere—in the house, in the garden, in the woods, and along the roadside. There are more than 700 species of plants known to cause illness and death, but few persons besides the trained botanist know which plants fall into that category. Attention is called here to a number of them.

Houseplants

Certain houseplants may be deadly if ingested. Daffodils, hyacinths, and narcissi will cause nausea, vomiting, and diarrhea, and even death. The leaves and branches of oleander contain a digitalis-like deadly heart stimulant so powerful that a single leaf if eaten may kill a child. It is reported that people have died merely from eating steaks that have been speared on oleander twigs and roasted over a fire. One leaf of poinsettia if eaten by a child causes death, as it contains a lethal acrid burning juice. Children have died after eating berries of the mistletoe; so have adults who drank tea made by brewing the berries. The stalk of *Dieffenbachia*, also known as "dumb cane" contains needle-like crystals of calcium oxalate that become embedded in the tissues of the mouth and tongue. If the base of the tongue becomes sufficiently enlarged to block air passage, death by suffocation may result. It derived its name of dumb cane because of its power to make it difficult or impossible for a person thus affected to speak due to the pain and swelling within the mouth.

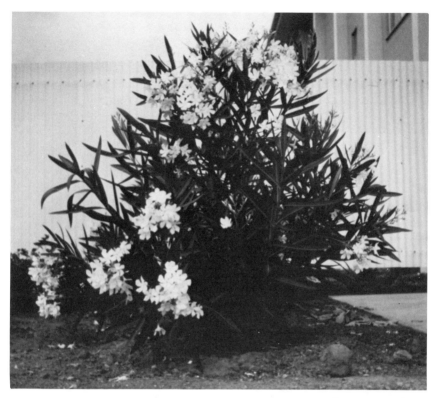

From Kingsbury (1964)
Reprinted by permission of Prentice-Hall, Inc.

FIG. 21.1. OLEANDER

Garden Plants

Among the garden plants that have been found to be poisonous are the seeds of larkspur, the fleshy roots of monkshood, the leaves and flowers of lily-of-the-valley, the autumn crocus bulb, the underground stem of iris, all the parts of azalea, and the leaves of foxglove (the source of the cardiac stimulant digitalis).

Berries from daphne, jessamine, lantana, and yews may prove lethal if eaten by a child. Mountain laurel was used by the Delaware Indians to make suicide potions. Seeds and pods of wisteria may cause digestive upset. Bees visiting rhododendron flowers produce a toxic honey. The seeds and leaves of jimson weed that grows everywhere, if eaten will cause stramonium poisoning with abnormal thirst, distorted sight, delirium, incoherence, and coma. Death has occurred among teenagers who

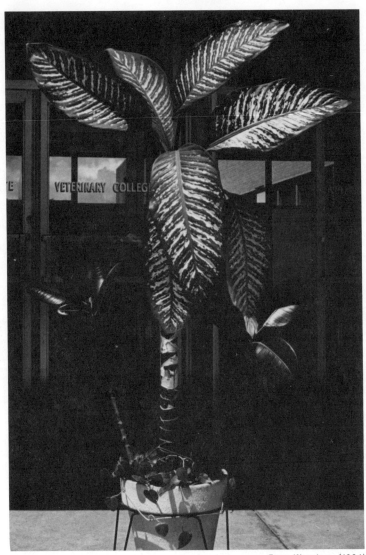

From Kingsbury (1964)
Reprinted by permission of Prentice-Hall, Inc.

FIG. 21.2. DUMB CANE

brewed jimson weed tea and drank it for "kicks." In some areas of the
South, tomato plants are grafted to the roots of jimson weed, thus producing larger and frost-resistant tomatoes. However, where the grafting
was made on a branch above the ground, poisoning occurred.

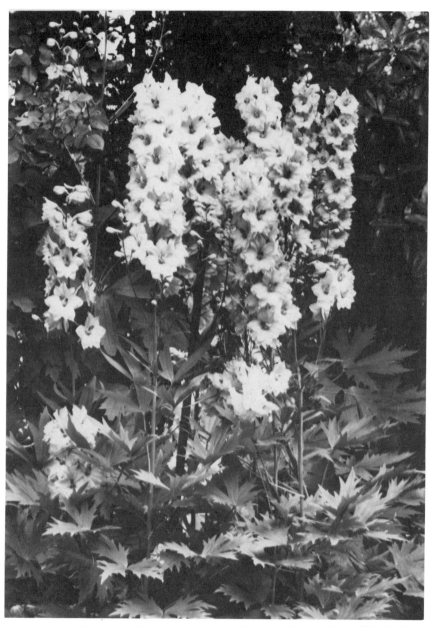

Courtesy of Library of the New York Botannical Garden, Bronx, N.Y., Mr. Seigel

FIG. 21.3. *DELPHINIUM* SP.

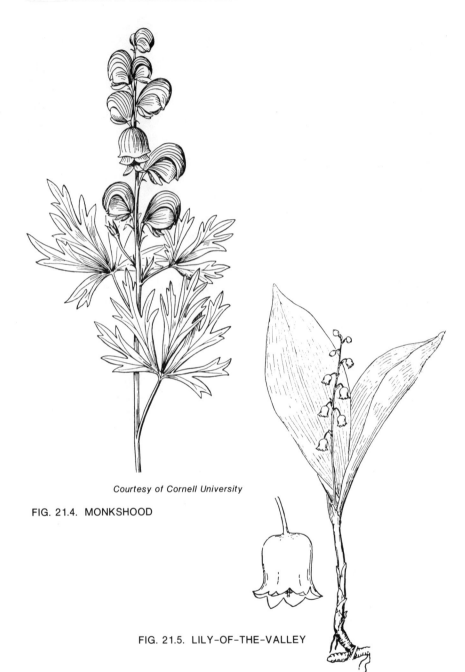

Courtesy of Cornell University

FIG. 21.4. MONKSHOOD

FIG. 21.5. LILY-OF-THE-VALLEY

Courtesy of Cornell University

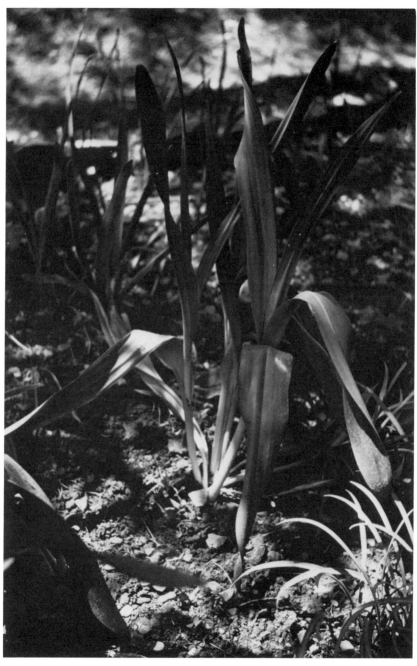

From Kingsbury (1964)
Reprinted by permission of Prentice-Hall, Inc.

FIG. 21.6. AUTUMN CROCUS

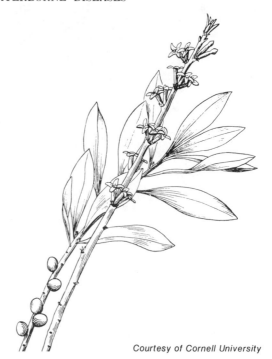

FIG. 21.7. DAPHNE

Courtesy of Cornell University

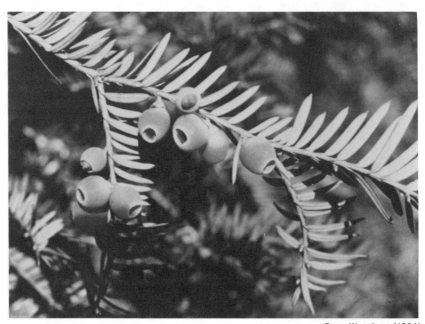

From Kingsbury (1964)
Reprinted by permission of Prentice-Hall, Inc.

FIG. 21.8. YEW

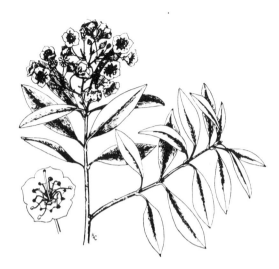

FIG. 21.9. MOUNTAIN
LAUREL

Courtesy of Cornell University

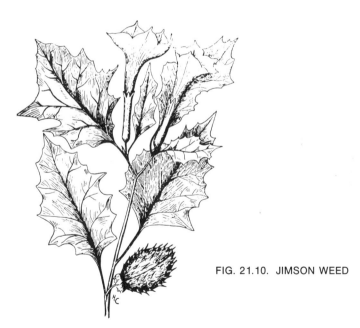

FIG. 21.10. JIMSON WEED

Courtesy of Cornell University

Field Plants

There are plants growing in the fields that should not be ingested.
Buttercups produce an irritating juice that causes gastroenteritis. Night-

shade, especially its unripe berries, results in intense digestive and nervous symptoms and may prove fatal. Poison hemlock, a potion of which killed the ancient Greek philosopher Socrates, as its title indicates, is extremely poisonous.

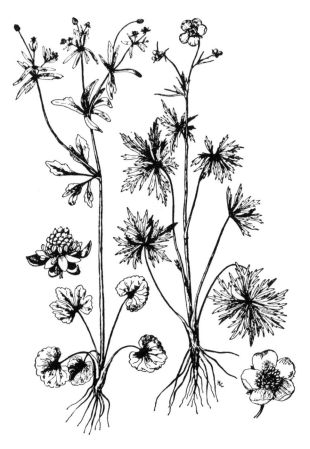

Courtesy of Cornell University

FIG. 21.11. LEFT—SMALL FLOWERED BUTTERCUP
RIGHT—TALL FIELD BUTTERCUP

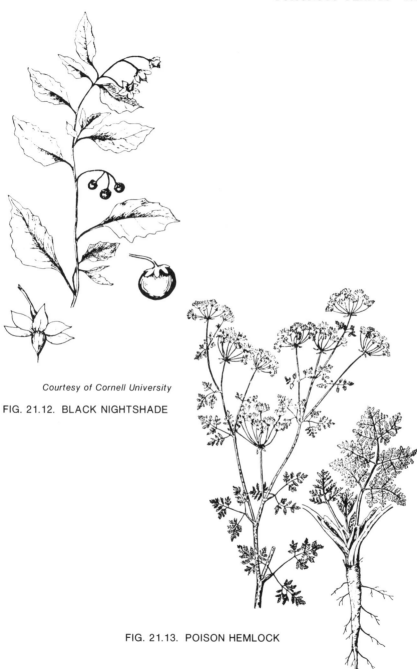

Courtesy of Cornell University

FIG. 21.12. BLACK NIGHTSHADE

FIG. 21.13. POISON HEMLOCK

Courtesy of Cornell University

Trees

Parts of fruit trees, other than the fruit they bear, should be avoided. Twigs and foliage of the cherry tree and the peach tree release cyanide if chewed or eaten, causing gasping, excitement, and prostration. Apricot kernels also contain cyanide and should not be eaten or brewed in hot water. Although acorns are a suitable food for squirrels, children are made ill with renal symptoms from chewing them. Children have also been made sick by using pieces of the pithy stems of elderberry for blowguns.

Berries and Seeds

Children have been poisoned, fatally in some instances, after eating brightly colored or unripe berries. Severe burns of the mouth and the digestive tract are caused by those of *Daphne mezereon*. Nightshade and *Lantana camara* berries are also toxic.

Rosary pea seeds have an attractive enamel red and black shell. They are made into necklaces and sold to tourists as souvenirs. A single seed, if chewed, may kill a child. Necklaces made with castor beans that resemble beetles contain recin, and may similarly prove lethal to a child.

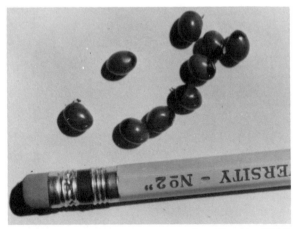

FIG. 21.14. ROSARY PEA SEEDS

From Kingsbury (1964)
Reprinted by permission of Prentice-Hall, Inc.

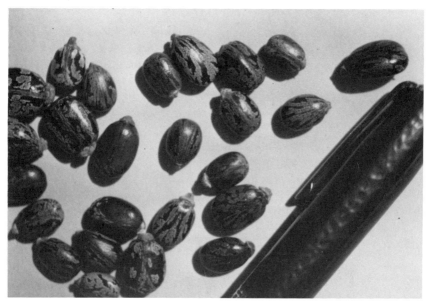

From Kingsbury (1964)
Reprinted by permission of Prentice-Hall, Inc.

FIG. 21.15. CASTOR BEAN SEEDS

Food Items

Even such staple items of food as potatoes and tomatoes come from plants related to the deadly nightshade. Although the tomato fruit and the potato tuber are edible, their foliage and vines contain an alkaloid poison that causes digestive and nervous disorders.

The stems of rhubarb are delectable, but the leaf blades contain 1% oxalic acid that may crystallize in the kidneys if eaten cooked or raw in large quantity and may cause convulsions and coma often followed by death. In 1961 toxicologists were astonished when they noted that the new edition of *Larousse Gastronomique* cookbook (Montagné 1961) stated that rhubarb leaves may be "eaten like spinach."

Prevention

Plant poisoning may be prevented by keeping all plants away from children who may nibble on them. Children should be taught never to eat or put in their mouths any plants or berries not used as food. Adults should refrain from making medicinal concoctions or teas from plants, and they should not chew plant stems.

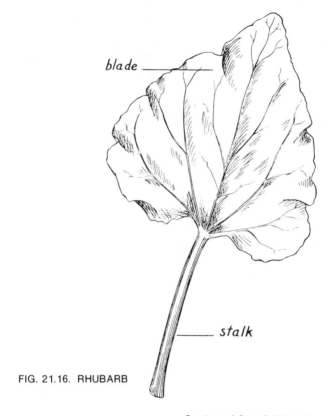

blade

stalk

FIG. 21.16.   RHUBARB

Courtesy of Cornell University

Treatment

If poisoning occurs, a physician or the Poison Control Center should be called. As with chemical poisoning, it is not always advisable to induce vomiting or perform gastric lavage, as some plants contain corrosive juices that may severely damage tissues of the digestive tract. In addition, the strain of vomiting and the passage of the stomach tube may further injure the tissues.

Case Histories

A study of 100 child poisonings in the Seattle area showed that nearly 10% of the youngsters had eaten toxic plants. In most of the instances, the children's parents had no idea that the plants were poisonous. Several reports of such poisonings are given below.

(1) Within hours after 30 boys, ages 6 to 8, returned from an orphan-age outing in the Midwest, complete pandemonium broke loose. Some children began to laugh senselessly, pick imaginary objects out of the air, and bark like dogs. Others crawled under their beds, crying and moaning. A visiting physician administered drugs to them and induced vomiting. The next day most of the boys return-ed to normal and all recovered completely in 3 days. On question-ing, the boys said they had found an abundant patch of what turn-ed out to be jimson weed and had playfully picked and eaten vary-ing amounts of it.

(2) In Ohio one summer, a little girl prepared a play luncheon in the back yard. She placed on a miniature plate an apple, a radish, and some red berries she had picked from a shrub growing in her mother's rock garden. Four hours later she lapsed into coma and 7 hours after the play luncheon she was dead. An autopsy showed that the berries she had eaten were from the daphne plant, the berries of which contain a corrosive poison.

(3) In Tacoma, Washington, a 3-year-old girl died suddenly and at first doctors thought she had choked on a piece of peppermint candy. Intensive investigation revealed that she was a victim of the fruit of the deadly nightshade bush that grew near her home.

(4) During 1961 and 1962, 2 physicians in Florida reported that they had treated 17 children for ingestion of the red berries of red sage. Four of the children were hospitalized with severe poisoning and 1 girl, age 2½, died several hours after eating the berries.

(5) Several children in New Jersey and in the South became ill after eating as few as 2 seeds of wisteria, a very common vine.

The drawings in this chapter are by Elfride Abbe and Helen Hill Craig.

REFERENCES

DEWBERRY, E.B. 1959. Food Poisoning. Leonard Hill, London.

GIBSON, R.K. 1961. Jimson weed poisoning in children. J. Indiana State Med. Assoc. *54*, 101.

HART, M. 1963. Hazards to health. Jequirity bean poisoning. N. Engl. J. Med. *268*, 886.

KINGSBURY, J.M. 1964. Poisonous Plants of the United States and Canada. Prentice-Hall, Englewood Cliffs, N.J. Photographs reprinted by permission, pp. 121, 195, 303, 450, 474.

KINGSBURY, J.M. 1976. Common poisonous plants. N.Y. State Coll. Agric. Life Sci., Cornell Univ. Inf. Bull. *104*.

LAMPE, K.F. and FAGERSTROM, R. 1968. Plant Toxicity and Dermatitis. Williams & Wilkins Co., Baltimore.

LARKIN, T. 1975. Natural poisons in food. FDA Consumer, Off. Public Affairs, Dep. Health, Educ. Welfare Publ. (FDA) 76-2009.

MELVILLE, A. and FASTIEV, F.N. 1964. Detection of certain honey poisons. Proc. Univ. Otago Med. Sch. 42, 3.

MONTAGNÉ, P. 1961. Larousse Gastronomique: The Encyclopedia of Food, Wine & Cookery. C. Turgeon and N. Froud (Editors). Crown Publishers, New York.

MUENSCHER, W.C. 1956. Poisonous Plants in the United States. Macmillan Co., New York.

NATL. RES. COUNC. 1973. Toxicants Occurring Naturally in Foods, 2nd Edition. National Academy of Sciences, Washington, D.C.

N.Y. STATE DEP. HEALTH. 1964. Poison in the Back Yard. Family Safety, Special Health Services, N.Y. State Dep. Health, Albany.

N.Y. STATE DEP. HEALTH. 1967. Safety council says poison plants are abundant. N.Y. State Dep. Health Bull. 20 (39) 155.

POTTER, N.N. 1978. Food Science, 3rd Edition. AVI Publishing Co., Westport, Conn.

SCHWARTING, A.E. 1963. Poisonous seeds and fruits. Prog. Chem. Toxicol. 1, 385.

SCOTT, H.C. 1969. Poisonous plants and animals. In Foodborne Infections and Intoxications. H. Riemann (Editor). Academic Press, New York.

YOUNGKEN, H.W., JR. and KARAS, J.S. 1964. Common poisonous plants of New England. U.S. Dep. Health, Educ. Welfare, Public Health Serv. Publ. 1230.

22

Natural Food Poisons

Let us suppose, just hypothetically, that an enterprising farmer contacted the Department of Agriculture or the Food and Drug Administration and informed the agency that he had succeeded in cultivating a vegetable crop that he believed would prove a nutritious item of food. He stated that he had fed it to his farm animals with no evidence of any deleterious result, and he would like the opinion of the agencies as to whether the vegetable was safe for humans to eat so that he could market it.

A representative of the agency would probably be dispatched to the farm to gather up several of the plants, (roots, stalks, and leaves) for examination by its botanists and food chemists. When the tests were completed, the farmer would be informed that the botanists had found the plant to be a member of the nightshade family, a poisonous plant capable of causing severe gastroenteritis and nervous disorders. The chemists had analyzed the vegetable part of the plant and found that it contained at least 150 different chemicals, among which were the following toxicants: (1) oxalic acid that when ingested interferes with the body's absorption of calcium; (2) tannin, a poisonous and possibly carcinogenic chemical; (3) nitrate, capable of causing severe gastroenteritis; (4) arsenic, a powerful poison; and (5) solanine, an alkaloid neurotoxin related to nerve gas that interferes with the transmission of nerve impulses.

Although these toxic chemicals are present in extremely small quantities, the agency feels that it can not approve this vegetable as a safe food for human consumption.

The vegetable in our hypothetical story is the lowly potato that has been used as a staple food by man for millennia. With the exception of the real hazard from solanine present in the skin of green potatoes and in the sprouts on stored potatoes, the other toxic products found on analysis are present in such minute quantities that they may be safely ignored.

Thomas Larkin, in 1975, as special assistant to the Commissioner of Food and Drugs stated:

Food is nothing more than an amalgam of chemicals, and some of the substances that occur naturally in the things we eat every day are potentially as lethal as Lucretia Borgia's favorite recipes. But in most instances the natural toxicants in food don't threaten our health because they are present in such small quantities that the protective mechanisms of the body can deal with them.

Some other foods that contain small quantities of toxic chemicals produced by nature are rhubarb and spinach that harbor oxalic acid; cabbage, brussels sprouts, soybean, mustard, and onion that contain goitrogens capable of causing goiter by blocking the body's ability to absorb adequate amounts of iodine; lima beans, peas, sweet potatoes, yams, cherries, and apricots that have chemicals related to cyanide; bananas that have pressure amines that can increase blood pressure but are held in check by an enzyme (monoamine oxidase); and coffee that has its caffeine. A number of spices contain safrol (from sassafras root) that in high concentration may cause cancer of the liver. It is fortunate that the toxicants in a number of foods are inactivated by heating.

It is obvious that it is impossible to completely avoid natural toxicants in foods. Although harmless in the concentrations in which they appear in food, they may prove hazardous if excessive quantities of any of the foods are consumed daily, as may be the case with some fad diets. The same may be said of certain additives put into food for the purpose of improving its taste or to prevent its spoilage.

To protect oneself against the undesirable action of natural food toxicants, one should eat a balanced diet and avoid concentrating on any one food. Remember that small amounts of poison may be tolerated but that large quantities are harmful.

One may speculate about whether some unexplained cases of illness in certain persons are due to their inability to tolerate even micro-doses of some of the natural toxicants in the foods they eat.

There are, however, some foods of animal and plant origin that under certain circumstances may contain toxicants in proportions large enough to cause severe illness, even death, when ingested. Mention has been made of honey that may prove poisonous when produced by bees that had collected pollen from rhododendron flowers (Chapter 21) and the poisonous nature of certain mushrooms has also been discussed (Chapter 19).

Milk Sickness

During the early part of the 19th century in the United States, early settlers in the Midwest, among them the mother of Abraham Lincoln, died of milk sickness, also known as "alkali poisoning." There were many outbreaks of the disease, some being so extensive as to be responsible for depopulating some villages. The cause of the outbreaks was traced to milk and milk products from cows that were permitted to forage on white snakeroot that contains a toxic constituent trematode, so named because the cows that produced the tainted milk suffered from what colloquially was called "the trembles." An outbreak of milk sickness with 21 cases and 2 deaths were reported in Illinois in 1938, and sporadic cases still occur. Pasteurization of such milk fails to destroy its poisonous property.

The symptoms of milk fever are excessive thirst, weakness, pernicious vomiting, severe constipation, epigastric pain, and prostration. In severe cases there are convulsions and coma followed by death.

Favism

There is a broad bean known as the fava bean *(Vicia fava)* that is a staple article of diet in Mediterranean countries. The beans are also grown in this country in the backyards of individuals of Italian descent. When ingested by persons who have been previously sensitized either by inhaling the pollen of the blossoms of the fava plant or by prior ingestion of the beans, severe illness may occur. It has been found that the first green beans of the season are the most poisonous. Toxicity is due to a nucleoside (vicine) that causes hemolysis when injected into rabbits.

Illness known as favism usually appears within 1 hr after ingestion, the patient complaining of dizziness, vomiting, diarrhea, and severe prostration followed by acute febrile anemia, jaundice, and hematuria (blood in the urine). Treatment is symptomatic with replacement of electrolytes and blood transfusion in severe cases.

Favism should be considered as a possible cause of hemolytic anemia in communities with large Italian populations, although favism has also been reported in other ethnic groups.

Legumes

Sweet peas, lima beans, kidney beans, navy beans, Jack beans, and soybeans, if eaten when insufficiently cooked, have been found to contain hemagglutinins capable of agglutinating red blood cells. This has been confirmed by animal feeding experiments.

Bracken

An apparently harmless fern, *Zen mai*, is used as a vegetable and a seasoning by the Japanese. However, another fern, bracken, is often confused with *Zen mai* and when eaten causes damage to the intestinal mucosa. When fed to rats, it produces multiple adenocarcinomas of the small intestine. This could account for the relatively high incidence of gastric cancer among the Japanese.

Other foods with carcinogenic properties in rats, causing cancer of the liver, are peanut meal attacked by mold, yellow moldy rice, and the antibiotic griseofulvin.

Seafood Poisoning

Between the months of June and October when the plankton *Gonyaulax* grows in such abundance that the waters of its habitat turn red in color, mussels that feed on these diatoms become poisonous. The reason is that the plankton contains a strong alkaloid so poisonous that a few milligrams, if ingested, may prove fatal within 5 to 30 min. Patients complain of respiratory paralysis, numbness, trembling about the mouth and lips, and complete loss of muscle power of the neck and extremities. Outbreaks of mussel poisoning were originally reported along the Pacific coast.

Certain fish are poisonous as they contain a naturally occurring neurotoxin. Ingestion of the flesh or liver of such fish may give rise to nausea, vomiting, diarrhea, abdominal pain, chills, fever, sweating, joint pains, circumoral tingling, numbness of the limbs, and painful urination. The incubation period varies from several minutes to 30 hr and the symptoms depend on the type of fish ingested.

Among the fish capable of causing ichthyosarcotoxism (fish poisoning) are (1) Caribbean type (sierra, cavallas, groupers, great barracuda, and amberjack)—this type of poisoning is nonfatal; (2) Pacific type (sea bass, trigger fish, black ulna, red snapper, barracuda, and eel), fatality rate of this type is about 3%; (3) *Tetraodon* type in Japanese waters (globe fish, baloon fish, and puffer)—this type has a fatality rate of 73%.

Scombroid fishes (tuna, bonito, mackerel, and skipjack) are not toxic when cooked immediately upon being caught; however, a poison is rapidly formed by bacterial action in the flesh following the death of the fish. Puffer fish flesh can be made edible by thorough washing when the fish has just been caught.

Eating the liver or certain portions of sharks, dogfish, or rays will cause nausea, vomiting, abdominal pain, oily feces, headache, tingling of the lips, tongue, and throat, visual disturbances, pain in the limbs, chest pain, coma, and even death.

It is said that the Chinese have a proverb that says, "Eat porpoise if you wish to discard life." It originated in 1883 when it was reported that 5 persons in Anch'ing that year and one in Yanchow in the following year died after eating portions of porpoise, a food highly esteemed in China. It was subsequently learned that porpoises that go far inland along the Yangtze become poisonous, probably because of eating some toxic food. Their blood, liver, fat, and entrails when eaten caused pain, marked swelling of the abdomen, cyanosis, swelling and numbness of the tongue, dimness of vision, and dribbling of greenish saliva from the mouth.

In Japan where 10% of the food supply is from marine organisms, poisoning by seafood is estimated to be responsible for 60 to 70% of all food poisoning. The preference of the Japanese for raw fish and their ingestion of cephalopods (squid and octopus) are contributory factors.

In a study of the period 1952–1955, although no death resulted, 21 persons became ill out of 210 who ate octopus. The predominant symptoms were gastrointestinal with mild fever, headache, chills, and weakness, with some patients developing paralysis or convulsions.

Prevention

No organisms known to be causative agents of any of the ordinary types of bacterial food infection appear to be responsible for the toxicity of the foods discussed, with the exception in the case of scombroid fish. The toxic substance contained in certain types of seafood depends on the presence of active material inside their gastrointestinal lumen. Toxicity often disappears rapidly following the emptying of their digestive tract. General rules for avoiding intoxication are:

(1) Do not eat the skin, liver, or gonads of fish.
(2) Soak flesh of suspected toxic fish in several changes of clear salted water before cooking.
(3) Cook fish immediately upon being caught. You must not depend on cooking to destroy all toxic substances.

Treatment

Treatment depends on how soon after ingestion it is started. If symptoms appear early, the contents of the stomach should be removed by lavage or by an emetic (ipecac syrup 4 to 8 ml orally every 15 min until vomiting is induced). If several hours have elapsed before treatment is started, gastric lavage and emetics are of no value as the offending agent will have left the stomach. Should vomiting persist and dehydration occur, fluids and electrolytes should be replaced parenterally.

Man through the ages has been able to determine only by trial and error which foods were safe to eat and which were poisonous by noting their effect on himself, his family, or his peers. Today, with our understanding of toxicology, with modern laboratory procedures, and animal experimentation, determination of poisonous or carcinogenic potentialities of foods may be made with a greater degree of certainty.

REFERENCES

ANDERSON, L.D. 1960. Toxic shellfish in British Columbia. Am. J. Public Health *51*, 71.

CAMPBELL, A.D. 1967. Natural food poisons. Food Drug Admin. (Sept.) 23.

COON, J.M. 1975. Natural toxicants in food. J. Am. Diet. Assoc. *67*, 213.

EDWARDS, H.T. 1956. The etiology and epidemiology of paralytic shellfish poisoning. J. Milk Food Technol. *19*, 331.

FOO, L.Y. 1977. Scombroid poisoning—Recapitulation on the role of histamine. N.Z. Med. J. *85*, 425.

GUDGER, E.W. 1930. Poisonous fishes and fish poisoning, with special references to Ciguatera in the West Indies. Am. J. Trop. Med. *10*, 45.

HALSTEAD, B.W. 1958. Poisonous fishes. Public Health Rep. *73*, 302.

HELFRICH, P. 1961. Fish Poisoning in the Tropical Pacific. Univ. of Hawaii Marine Laboratory, Honolulu.

HUGHES, J.M. and MERSON, M.H. 1976. Fish and shellfish poisoning. N. Engl. J. Med. *295*, 1117.

JENSSEN, W.A. 1970. Fish as potential vector of human bacterial disease. *In* A Symposium on Diseases of Fish and Shellfish. S.F. Sniezko (Editor). Spec. Publ. *5*. American Fisheries Society, Washington, D.C.

KAWABATA, T. 1962. Fish-borne poisoning in Japan. *In* Fish as Food, Vol. 2. G. Borgstrom (Editor). Academic Press, N.Y.

LARKIN, T. 1975. Natural Poisons in Food. U.S. Public Health Serv., U.S. Dep. Health, Educ. Welfare (PDA) *76–2009*.

MACGOWAN, D.J. 1883. Report on the Health of Wenchow for the Half-year Ending 30th September 1883. Chin. Imp. Marine Customs, Med. Rep., 26th Issue, Statistical Dep., Inspectorate Gen. Customs, Shanghai (porpoise poisoning).

MACGOWAN, D.J. 1884. Report on the Health of Wenchow for the Half-year Ending 31st March 1884. Chin. Imp. Marine Customs, Med. Rep., 27th Issue, Statistical Dep., Inspectorate Gen. Customs, Shanghai (porpoise poisoning.)

McCARTHY, O.R. 1955. A case of favism. Lancet *1*, 748.

MERCK AND CO. 1977. The Merck Manual of Diagnosis and Therapy, 13th Edition. Merck, Sharp and Dohme Research Laboratories, Division of Merck and Co., Rahway, N.J.

MONRO, I.C. 1976. Natural occurring toxicants in food and their significance. Clin. Toxicol. *9*, 647.

NATL. ACAD. SCI. NATL. RES. COUNC. 1966. Toxicants occurring naturally in foods. Natl. Acad. Sci., Natl. Res. Counc. Publ. *1354*.

ROTH, K.L. and FRUMIN, A.M. 1960. Studies on the hemolytic principle of the fava bean. J. Lab. Clin. Med. *56*, 695.

SHUBIK, P. and HARTWELL, J.L. 1959. Survey of compounds which have been tested for carcinogenic activity. U.S. Dep. Health, Educ. Welfare, U.S. Public Health Serv. Publ. *149*, Supplement 1.

23

Prevention of Foodborne Diseases

It is common knowledge that foods as a class are perishable. Meats begin to deteriorate shortly after slaughter; fish start spoiling promptly as soon as removed from their natural habitat; fruits and vegetables become impaired after harvesting. Pathogenic microorganisms such as *Salmonella* may be naturally found in such foods as eggs, poultry, and red meats; *Bacillus cereus* is a part of the normal flora of grains and cereals. It is therefore of utmost importance that foods be handled, processed, and stored in such a manner as to not promote further spoilage, to prevent multiplication of any organisms the food may contain, and to preclude the additional introduction of pathogenic agents.

Control measures for foods susceptible to such contamination involve: (1) sanitary methods in their handling; (2) the application of heat to destroy any living organisms that may be present; and (3) refrigeration at adequate low temperature to arrest microbial growth.

Sanitation

All the principles of sanitation must be carried out by persons engaged in the handling of food. Studies have shown that 50 to 60% of the normal population carry coagulase-positive staphylococci on their skin and in their nasopharynx, and that about 90% of the feces of normal persons contain *Clostridium perfringens*. The soil serves as a habitat for *C. botulinum* types A and B and for the eggs and ova of a number of intestinal parasites.

It is a fact that the majority of foodborne outbreaks are due to the unsanitary handling of food. There is no doubt that a considerable number of cases of gastroenteritis would have been avoided if the persons who prepared or served the incriminated foods had taken the trouble to wash their hands thoroughly after the use of the toilet before handling the foods. Individuals with skin infections, upper respiratory infections, or gastroenteritis should refrain from preparing food.

Heat

Although cooking cannot be relied upon to destroy toxins and chemicals responsible for food poisoning, it will destroy pathogenic organisms present in food. In adequate cooking, the center of the food should attain a temperature of 73.9° to 76.6°C (165° to 170°F). Leftover food should be reheated to at least 73.9°C (165°F) before it is served. Foods held on steam tables should be kept at 60°C (140°F) or above. When serving or slicing cooked meats or chicken, never do so on a table where uncooked meats have been placed.

Refrigeration

Every foodhandling establishment must have adequate refrigeration facilities so that perishable foods may be stored in the range of 0.0° to 4.4°C (32° to 40°F) in order to prevent the growth and toxin production of organisms capable of causing illness. Foods should not be kept at temperatures between 7.2°C and 60°C (45° and 140°F), as the incubation and multiplication of pathogens are favored at that range. Foods should be refrigerated as promptly as possible after their preparation. If food is to be frozen, its center must be reduced to a temperature of −32°C (0°F) or lower.

Foods at Parties

Luncheons or suppers prepared and served by members of fraternal groups, societies, churches, and other organizations have, on occasion, resulted in outbreaks of vomiting and purging among the guests who partook of the foods. The persons in charge and those who volunteered in the preparation of the refreshments can prevent such unpleasant occurrences by following these simple steps:

(1) *Water*: Use water of sanitary quality from a safe municipal supply.
(2) *Milk*: Use only pasteurized milk and cream for drinking and in the preparation of food.
(3) *Foods*: Avoid preparing and serving moist bland foods in which bacteria readily grow, such as macaroni, spaghetti, turkey and chicken stuffing, gravies, salads, custards, creamed dishes, and custard-filled pastries. These foods are nutritious and inexpensive and may be served only if prepared immediately before serving so

that they are not exposed to room temperature for any prolonged period of time.

(4) *Storage and Refrigeration*: If prepared food is to be stored and served later, it must be rapidly cooled and refrigerated until just before serving, then made hot (not warm) when it is served. Pouring hot sauce over cool meats is unsatisfactory. Regrettably many churches and organizations do not have well-equipped cooking, storage, and refrigeration facilities. For that reason, volunteers usually prepare the foods in their own kitchens and take it cooked to the gathering. These foods should then be refrigerated to temperatures below 7.2°C (45°F). Prepared foods should not be stored in "cool" church basements.

(5) *Volunteers*: Members who have a cold, cough, diarrhea, or any skin infection should not volunteer to prepare any food.

(6) *Serving*: The most satisfactory and safest procedure is to serve foods as soon as they are prepared. They should go directly from the stove or oven to the table. If at all possible, the foods should be prepared on the premises where the gathering is held.

(7) *Washing and Sanitizing*: Washing and sanitizing tableware, utensils, and equipment is an important step in controlling contamination. If the area where food is to be served for parties lacks the facilities for proper cleaning and sanitizing of tableware and utensils, the use of single-service disposable tableware is recommended.

Caterers

Caterers who provide food and services for social gatherings should follow the same principles of sanitation as food processors. They should use high quality ingredients and minimize human contact in their preparations. They must separate raw and finished products. Foods must be protected against environmental contamination. Refrigeration of prepared foods is of the utmost importance in their storage and transportation to the place where they are to be served, particularly during the summer months. Extreme care must be taken in the preparation and serving of foods that support microbial growth, such as fowl, turkey, beef and pork, milk and milk products, and shellfish.

The following two chapters on the food processing and the food service industries discuss preventive measures that apply to those phases of food commercialism. It is hoped that readers professionally engaged in those branches of food production and handling will benefit from the information imparted in those chapters.

REFERENCES

BANWART, G.J. 1979. Basic Food Microbiology. AVI Publishing Co., West-port, Conn.

BENENSON, A.S. 1975. Control of Communicable Diseases in Man, 12th Edition. Am. Public Health Assoc., Washington, D.C.

BRYAN, F.L. and McKINLEY, T.W. 1974. Prevention of foodborne illness by time-temperature control of thawing, cooking, chilling and reheating turkeys in school lunch kitchens. J. Milk Food Technol. 37, 420.

GUTHRIE, R.K. 1972. Food Sanitation. AVI Publishing Co., Westport, Conn.

LONGRÉE, K. 1968. Quality Food Sanitation. Interstate Publishers, Division of John Wiley & Sons, New York.

U.S. DEP. HEALTH, EDUC. WELFARE. 1971. Workshop 1—Prevention of contamination of raw agricultural and marine products. *In* Proc. 1971 Natl. Conf. Food Protection, Denver, 1971. U.S. Dep. Health, Educ. Welfare, U.S. Govt. Printing Off., Washington, D.C.

U.S. DEP. HEALTH, EDUC. WELFARE, PUBLIC HEALTH SERV. 1958. Epidemiology and Control of Foodborne Disease. U.S. Govt. Printing Off., Washington, D.C.

24

Commercial Food Processing

Rufus K. Guthrie and his collaborators (1972) in their book *Food Sanitation* give an excellent description of sanitation as it applies to the commercial production, processing, and service of foods. Workers in the food industry and persons engaged in the operation of public eating establishments will greatly benefit from the recommendations enumerated in the book for the protection of the public health and the prevention of gastrointestinal illness. It must be emphasized that food sanitation is not only an economic asset to the industry, it is as well an economic and health necessity to the consumers.

In addition, it is advisable for supervising personnel in the food industry not to hesitate to avail themselves of the services of public health representatives such as epidemiologists, sanitary engineers, and sanitarians as consultants in the following areas:

(1) Individual and group instruction of management in the nature and control of foodborne diseases, and their responsibilities in this matter.
(2) Consultation and advice on sanitary operating procedures.
(3) Consultation on business practice as it relates to communicable disease control.
(4) Consultation and advice on sanitary maintenance through supervisory practices in the establishment.
(5) Field tests of equipment, procedures, and materials.
(6) Organization of all available community resources to assist in food establishment sanitation improvement.

Food Processing Plant Equipment Sanitization

Since the cleaning operation is one of the principal prerequisities for maintaining sanitary control in food processing plants, the plant manager or his quality control personnel should study the various methods of cleaning and sanitizing equipment and select the one best suited to their particular operation. Plants where the equipment is suited to in-place cleaning, such as milk plants, carbonated beverage plants, and other similar plants, the appropriate personnel should study the system chosen, the detergents and sanitizing agents recommended, and make certain that every food contact surface of the equipment is subjected to rinsing, cleaning, and sanitizing. There should be no residues left after the completion of the cleaning operation.

If the food equipment is manually cleaned by a system known as out-of-place cleaning, the rinse water, cleaning solution, the concentration of the detergent, and the velocity of the circulating fluid should be designed for the type of operation depending upon the soiled condition of the equipment.

In order that food equipment may be adequately cleaned, it should be designed to be easily dismantled, be of smooth construction, devoid of crevices, be resistant to detergents, and be non-toxic.

Selection of Equipment.—To guide food plant operators and quality control personnel in their selection of equipment, the Dairy and Food Industry Equipment Committee of the New York State Association of Milk and Food Sanitarians has listed the following sources of equipment and their standards:

Address
The American Society of Mechanical Engineers
United Engineering Center, 345 E. 47th St., New York, NY 10017
Application of Standards
Provides acceptable design, manufacturing, and equipment standards for the production, preparation, and service of foods, drugs, and beverages where there are no recognized standards. It deals with sanitation, safety, contamination, and noise.

Address
Baking Industry Sanitation Standards Committee
521 Fifth Ave., New York, NY 10017
Application of Standards
Develops, approves, and publishes standards for sanitary design and construction of bakery machinery and equipment.

Address
National Automatic Merchandising Association
7 S. Dearborn St., Chicago, IL 60603

Application of Standards
Provides machine sanitary design and construction including safety and testing provisions for automatic food and beverage equipment. In addition, all food contact surfaces used in vending machines under NAMA Vending Machine Evaluation Program must meet FDA criterion.

Address
National Sanitation Foundation
NSF Building, Ann Arbor, MI 48105
  Application of Standards
  Establishes standards for food-service equipment, processes and products. It incorporates testing procedures and field inspections.

Address
Equipment Group, Technical Services, Meat Poultry Inspection Program (MPIP), Food Safety Quality Service (FSQS): U.S. Dep. Agric. (USDA) Washington, D.C. 20250
  Application of Standards
  Provides criteria for construction of equipment used in federally inspected meat and poultry plants.

Address
3-A Sanitary Standards Committee
Room 1050, 5530 Wisconsin Ave., Washington, D.C. 20015
  Application of Standards
  Provides sanitary standards and accepted practices for dairy and dairy product equipment.

Address
Poultry and Egg Institute of America
P.O. Box 9446, Rosslyn Station, Arlington, VA 22209
  Application of Standards
  Provides criteria for the sanitary construction of egg product processing equipment.

It should be borne in mind that with the purchase of equipment for which standards have been established, if installed in such a manner as to prevent easy access for dismantling and cleaning, the efficiency of that equipment will be greatly reduced.

Training and Resource Material

There is a vast store of literature for use in the training of sanitarians, persons in charge of quality control, and personnel in food processing plants in the proper utilization of equipment and its sanitary upkeep. Most trade organizations have programs for training their membership. Book publishing houses list a number of topics on food sanitation. The National Sanitation Foundation has developed educational material with visual aids which could be used effectively. The Journal of Food Protection published by the International Association of Milk, Food, and Environmental Sanitarians is an excellent source of information. The Food and Drug Administration, the U.S. Department of Agriculture, state colleges, and state agricultural and health departments publish resource material which could be used effectively. In reality, there is an ample supply of material for training courses on food production, processing, and food service sanitation. What is needed is the willingness to promote such programs.

REFERENCES

DESROSIER, N.W. and DESROSIER, J.N. 1977. The Technology of Food Preservation, 4th Edition. AVI Publishing Co., Westport, Conn.

GUTHRIE, R.K. 1972. Food Sanitation. AVI Publishing Co., Westport, Conn.

N.Y. STATE ASSOC. MILK FOOD SANITARIANS. 1975. Annual Report of Dairy and Food Industry Equipment Committee, Vol. 22. N.Y. State Assoc. of Milk and Food Sanitarians, Ithaca.

N.Y. STATE ASSOC. MILK FOOD SANITARIANS. 1978. Food Equipment Standards Chart. N.Y. State Assoc. of Milk and Food Sanitarians, Ithaca.

PARKER, M.E. and LICHFELD, J.H. 1962. Food Plant Sanitation. Reinheld Publishing Corp., New York.

U.S. DEP. HEALTH, EDUC. WELFARE, PUBLIC HEALTH SERV. 1958. Epidemiology and Control of Food-borne Disease. U.S. Govt. Printing Office, Washington, D.C.

U.S. DEP. HEALTH, EDUC. WELFARE. 1971. Workshop 2—Prevention of contamination of commercially processed foods. In Proc. 1971 Natl. Conf. Food Protection, Denver, 1971. U.S. Dep. Health, Educ. Welfare, U.S. Govt. Printing Off., Washington, D.C.

WEISER, H.H., MOUNTNEY, G.J. and GOULD, W.A. 1971. Practical Food Microbiology and Technology, 2nd Edition. AVI Publishing Co., Westport, Conn.

25

Food Service Establishments

During the past few decades, there has been a great change in the eating habits of the population of this country. The number of persons who eat one or more meals each day in public or private eating establishments has been growing steadily as more and more people are living in homes remote from their place of employment. An ever-growing number of women are joining the work force. A study by the U.S. Department of Commerce (1979) revealed that expenditure for food away from home increased from one-quarter of the food budget in 1957 to more than one-third of an approximately $200 billion food budget in 1977. Between 1965 and 1976 fast food establishments increased their share of away-from-home food expenditures from 10 to 25%. As a result, the food and beverage production and service industry ranks fourth in size among the industries in the nation and employs more people than any other industry.

Categories of Food Service Establishments

The Food and Drug Administration in its bulletin *Food Service Sanitation Manual* (U.S. Dep. Health, Educ. Welfare, Public Health Serv., Food Drug Admin. 1976) divides food service establishments into 4 categories depending upon the service rendered:

(1) Establishments open to public patronage, such as restaurants, cafes, cafeterias, fast-food outlets, luncheonettes, soda fountains, taverns, bars, hotels, drink-ins, mobile food and drink units, and food caterers. These constitute the major portion of the food service industry.
(2) Establishments offering semipublic food service to persons to whom other eating facilities are not available such as hospitals and related medical care institutions, schools and universities, employees' cafe-

terias, large department stores, penal institutions, and industrial plants.

(3) Establishments providing a limited type of food service such as private clubs, fraternal orders, various societies, churches, and religious affiliated organizations.

(4) Temporary food service establishments; these may not have adequate sanitary facilities such as permanent water supply, toilet and sewage system connection, and practical fixtures for the preparation and storage of foods.

Not only have food service establishments increased in size, number, and kind, but techniques in preparation and distribution have changed as evidenced by the trend toward industrial catering and centralized preparation. Food prepared in a single kitchen may serve large numbers of persons in plants, schools, airplanes, trains, hospitals, and other institutions. These changes, in turn, have created conditions whereby food processing, distribution and service need critical examination.

PREVENTION OF ILLNESS

George J. Banwart in *Basic Food Microbiology* (1979) states: "Due to large-scale, high-speed food processing, alteration of traditional methods resulting in less control of microorganisms, proliferation of heat-and-eat convenience foods and its nationwide distribution with increased potential for mishandling, there is concern that outbreaks of foodborne illness can occur that could involve very large numbers of people. The number of cases fluctuates from year to year but the number of cases per 100,000 people has tended to increase since 1967." Better reporting by regulatory agencies may account for part of the increase, but it may also be due to an actual increase in the number of cases.

In order to prevent the occurrence of gastrointestinal illness in the consuming public, the food service establishments must at all times protect the food they dispense against contamination with pathogenic microorganisms, chemicals, dust, vermin, and other noxious products. Food processors who supply these establishments must use only approved food additives and packaging material.

Food should be prepared in a clean, sanitary environment with adequate modern storage and refrigeration equipment, and persons involved in its preparation and service should be free of any transmissible disease.

If prepared food is to be transported for short or long distances, it must be placed in containers that will protect it from contamination, and proper temperature of the food must be maintained at all times during transportation. Operators in the food industry should depend upon good sanitation rather than on good luck.

Inspection of Service-food Establishments

The Food and Drug Administration requires a minimum of one inspection of each service-food establishment annually by an authorized representative of a regulatory agency to ascertain that no unsanitary condition exists which may constitute a danger to the public health. Some state and county regulatory agencies require more than one yearly inspection. The frequency of inspection should be based on the sanitary level of the industry involved. Should any violation be noted, corrective measures should be taken immediately.

In conducting a sanitary survey of the facilities of an establishment involved in serving food to the public, a number of basic conditions should be thoroughly checked:

(1) Food shall be from an approved source, wholesome and unadulterated. Special consideration should be given to foods classified as "potentially hazardous" as to their source, preparation, method of transportation, and display. The Food and Drug Administration *Food Service Sanitation Manual* (U.S. Dep. Health, Educ. Welfare, Public Health Serv., Food Drug Admin. 1976) defines potentially hazardous food to mean "any food that consists in whole or in part of milk and milk products, eggs, meat, poultry, fish, shellfish, edible crustacea, or other ingredients, including synthetic ingredients, in a form capable of supporting rapid and progressive growth of infectious or toxigenic microorganisms. The term does not include clean, whole, uncracked, odorfree shell fish, eggs or foods which have a pH level of 4.6 or below or a water activity (a_w) value of 0.85 or less."

Fresh and frozen shucked shellfish (oysters, clams, or mussels) shall be packed in nonreturnable packages identified with the name and address of the original shell stock processor, shucker-packer, or repacker, and the certification number. This is essential in tracing the source of the product in the event of a foodborne outbreak. The quality control personnel of a food processing plant should check not only incoming food to be processed, but should also, in cooperation with management, devise a system whereby identification of the product can be traced as to the date and time of manufacture, the unit and lot number, the number of the equipment used, and the plant number.

(2) Potentially hazardous food shall meet applicable temperature requirements during storage, preparation, display, service, and transportation. Foods requiring refrigeration after preparation shall be cooled to an internal temperature of 7.2°C (45°F) or below. When prepared in large volume or in large quantities, they shall be

rapidly cooled, utilizing such methods as shallow pans, agitation, quick chilling, or water circulation external to the food container so that the cooling period shall not exceed 4 hr. If transported, the food shall be prechilled and held at a temperature of 7.2°C (45°F) or below.

Gross violations occur frequently in retail outlets where the frozen food items are left standing without refrigeration. Although there may not be any appreciable growth of microorganisms in the food, there is a definite deterioration of nutritional value of such exposed food.

Ice used for cooling stored food and food containers shall not be used for human consumption.

The temperature of hot foods stored in bain-maries, steam tables, and steam kettles, or any other approved device used to maintain hot food, shall not be less than 60°C (140°F). Bain-maries and steam tables shall not be used for heating cold food.

(3) Potentially hazardous food once served shall not be reserved. Non-potentially hazardous food still packaged and in sound condition may be reserved.

(4) Toxic items shall be properly stored, labeled, and used. Poisonous or toxic materials consist of the following categories: insecticides and rodenticides; detergents, sanitizers, and related cleaning or drying agents; caustic acids, polishes, and other chemicals. Each of the categories shall be stored and physically located separate from each other. They shall not be stored above food or food equipment.

(5) Personnel with infections transmissible through food shall be restricted from food handling in food establishments. Persons who prepare or serve food shall maintain personal cleanliness and conform to good hygienic practices. It is the employer's responsibility to see that all employees connected with food preparation, service, or handling food equipment are in good health.

(6) Water supply shall be adequate, of safe and sanitary quality, and from an acceptable or approved source. Hot and cold running water under pressure shall be provided in all areas in the food establishment where the regulatory authorities deem it necessary for the safe and sanitary operation of the food establishment.

Lavatory facilities provided with hot and cold running water and liquid or powdered soap shall be provided in the kitchen and other food preparation areas for the use of employees.

(7) Sewage shall be disposed of in an acceptable or approved manner.

(8) Potable water system, plumbing, and equipment connected thereto shall be installed to preclude possibility of backflow.

(9) Effective measures shall be taken to protect against the entrance into the food establishment and the breeding or presence on the premises of insects and rodents.

(10) An effective method of breaking the chain of contamination in food service or in the food processing plant is to see that the equipment and utensils used to dispense or process food are clean visually and bacteriologically. Cleaning and sanitizing equipment must comply with recommended procedures. In order to be consistent with generally accepted practices, the recommendations of the Food and Drug Administration are listed as follows:

(a) *For Manual Cleaning, Rinsing, and Sanitizing* food service utensils and equipment, a 3-compartment sink is required. It shall be large enough to accommodate the equipment and utensils. Each compartment shall be supplied with hot and cold potable water (Fig. 25.1).

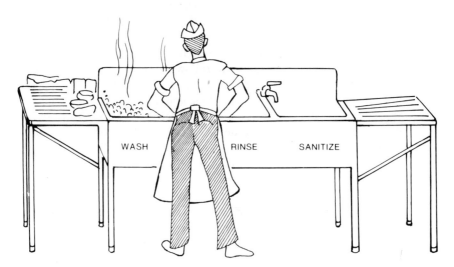

Courtesy of Nassau County Department of Health

FIG. 25.1. 3-COMPARTMENT SINK

Drain boards of adequate size shall be provided for proper handling of soiled utensils prior to washing and for cleaned utensils following sanitizing and shall be located so as not to interfere with the proper use of the dishwashing facilities.

Soiled equipment and utensils shall be pre-rinsed before washing.

Equipment and utensils shall be thoroughly washed in the first compartment with a hot detergent solution that is kept clean. They shall be rinsed free of detergent and abrasives with clear water in the second compartment, and sanitized in the third compartment in one of the following ways: (1) immersion for at least 0.5 min in clean, hot water at a temperature of at least 76.6°C (170°F); or (2) immersion for at least 1 min in a clean solution containing at least 50 ppm of available chlorine as a hypochlorite and at a temperature of at least 23.8°C (75°F); or (3) immersion for at least 1 min in a clear solution containing at least 12.5 ppm of available iodine and having a pH not higher than 5.0 and a temperature of at least 23.8°C (75°F).

Treatment with steam free from materials or additives is permitted.

Rinsing, spraying, or swabbing by chemical sanitizing solution twice the strength normally required shall be used in the case of equipment too large to sanitize by immersion.

To maintain the temperature when sanitizing, a heating device shall be provided under the sink. Dish baskets of such size and design as to permit complete immersion of the tableware and utensils in the hot water shall be used. When chemical sanitizers are used, a test kit is required for testing the concentration of the chemical used.

The 3-compartment sink with facilities as described can provide safety by removing the residue, making the utensils visibly and bacteriologically clean. It is well suited to small operations. However, experience shows that dishes, tableware, and glasses washed in this manner are not always bacteriologically clean.

Society considers dishwashing among the lowest types of manual labor. Usually the dishwasher is a person with little education and lacking other skills. The important social function he performs by preventing the transfer of pathogenic organisms through utensils is overlooked. Because of his lack of knowledge, in many cases he will be satisfied with his performance if he sees that utensils and tableware look clean. It is the responsibility of the owner to make him aware of his responsibility and he should be under constant supervision.

(b) *Dishwashing and Sanitizing by Machine in Food Service Establishments*: Mechanical cleaning and sanitizing may be done by spray-type or immersion dishwashing machines or any other type of machine or device that thoroughly cleans and sanitizes equipment and utensils. They shall be properly installed, maintained in good condition, and operated in accordance with manufacturers' instructions. Utensils placed in the machine shall be exposed to all dishwashing cycles.

Automatic detergent dispensers and wetting agent devices, if any, shall be properly installed and maintained.

The pressure of final rinse water in spray-type dishwashing machines shall not be less than 103.5 (15) nor more than 172.5 kPa (25 psi).

Accurate thermometers shall be provided to indicate the temperature of the water in each tank of the machine.

Drain boards shall be provided and be of adequate size for the proper handling of soiled utensils prior to washing and of cleaned utensils following sanitization.

Equipment and utensils shall be flushed or scraped and, when necessary, soaked prior to washing, after which they shall be air dried.

HANDLING OF FOOD IN SERVICE ESTABLISHMENTS

Food sanitation has made great strides during the final quarter of this century in the areas of refrigeration; in the sanitary design of equipment; in formulating regulations for sanitary operation and control of meat, milk and milk products, poultry products, shellfish, and other potentially hazardous foods; and in the food service operation.

Progress has been made possible because of: (1) the design and construction of mechanical refrigerators of different sizes for different functions; (2) the improvement in sanitary design of food processing and serving equipment; (3) the production of mechanical devices for controlling the proper operation of equipment such as that used in high-temperature-short-time milk pasteurizing; and (4) the formulation of new detergents and detergent sanitizers.

Despite advances in technology and extensive efforts to improve sanitary conditions and handling practices, food service workers continue to violate the basic principles of food protecton with the result that foodborne illness outbreaks have not substantially decreased.

Table 25.1 contains a compilation of foodborne disease outbreaks for 1977 as reported by the Center for Disease Control and a tabulation of the data (U.S. Dep. Health, Educ. Welfare, Public Health Serv., Cent. Dis. Control).

The data in Table 25.1 indicate that the food processing establishment (A) was responsible for only 1.8% of the total number of foodborne disease outbreaks. Each outbreak involved an average of 42 people. The

TABLE 25.1. FOODBORNE DISEASE OUTBREAKS, 1977

Location[1]	No. of Outbreaks	No. of Cases	No. of Cases per Outbreak	% of Outbreaks	% of Cases
A	8	342	42	1.8	3.6
B	287	6971	24	66.1	74.2
C	95	968	10	21.9	10.3
D	39	1084	27	8.9	11.5
E	5	28	5	1.1	0.3

[1]Location where the food was mishandled:
A—Food processing establishment.
B—Food service establishment.
C—Home.
D—Unknown.
E—Not applicable.

food service establishment (B) showed the highest incidence of the total number of outbreaks with 66.1%, but each outbreak involved an average of 24 persons. The percentage of cases attributed to outbreaks in the home (C) was 21.9% with each outbreak involving an average of 10 people. It was found, however, that of the 95 outbreaks with 968 cases which were alleged to have occurred in homes, 34 of the outbreaks with 273 cases occurred because of mishandling of the food before it was brought to the homes to be eaten.

The table reveals the critical areas to be the food service establishment and the home. However important this information is, it should not be overlooked that the outbreaks caused at the food processing establishments, though small in number, could involve a large number of people, cover an extensive area, and could be explosive in nature. It also, in all probability, would involve more than one jurisdiction. In reviewing the cases occurring at home, it should again be noted that an appreciable percentage of foods implicated and served at home were prepared and mishandled in food serving establishments or in food plants. Thus, the general criticism that the homemaker is negligent in his or her sanitary practices should not be overemphasized.

Many panel discussions have been held to look into the problem of mishandling of foods in commercial and institutional food service operations. The most outstanding was a panel on food protection held in Denver in April of 1971. Their immediate recommendations were:

(1) The adoption of uniform minimum laws, ordinances, and regulations by all states and communities engaged in regulating food service sanitation.
(2) Each inspecting agency should inform each food service operator of the applicable laws and the penalties for noncompliance.
(3) Enforcement agencies should identify critical operational food protection deficiencies, especially those causing most foodborne

illness outbreaks in food service establishments. Inspections must emphasize these deficiencies and the elimination of the hazards involved.

(4) The Food and Drug Administration should hold regional workshops to assist in the uniform interpretaton of regulations.

(5) Encourage food service operators to practice self-inspection, and provide them with instructional material.

(6) FDA should establish a clearinghouse for collecting and disseminating information on the sanitary control of potentially hazardous foods being shipped in interstate commerce. The FDA should convene a working committee of state and local regulatory officials and industry officials to establish guidelines, policies, and procedures for such a clearinghouse program.

The panel's long-range recommendations were that:

(1) The FDA establish an advisory committee composed of selected state, local, institutional, educational, and industry representatives (a) to develop a model industry self-inspection program; (b) to identify research needed to resolve current and emerging health problems associated with the preparation, display, storage, transportation, and service of foods in commercial and institutional food service operations; (c) to develop a detailed classification of potentially hazardous foods according to risk; (d) to evaluate and make recommendations to FDA as to the adequacy of its current resources and activities relating to the providing of technical and consultative assistance to states, communities, and the industry on food service sanitation.

(2) A system be developed and provisions introduced into food service establishment sanitation regulations and codes that require an establishment licensee and/or operating manager to demonstrate that he possesses the minimum essential knowledge of safe food handling and food protection practices.

(3) Consideration be given to the development of a model food protection study course for inclusion in all public and private secondary and vocational schools, with procedures for implementing its use by school administration; develop a self-study course on improving skills of personnel already employed in the food service industry.

(4) A study designed to evaluate traditional state and local programs as to their effectiveness be made by an agency outside of government.

(5) Each regulatory official be required to demonstrate that he understands principles of microbiology applicable to foodborne diseases.

For years the U.S. Public Health Service and presently the FDA have formulated model codes for inspection of the food service operation, yet there are many municipalities and states that have not adopted these codes. The Denver Food Protection Conference in 1971, sponsored by the Food and Drug Administration and organized by the American Public Health Association, emphasized the need for an interim code (U.S. Dep. Health, Educ. Welfare 1971). It has taken A.P.H.A. 8 years to ask its organization to promote the uniform code concept.

The need for reorganizing food protection activities on federal, state, and municipal levels is urgent if there is to be a reduction in the incidence of foodborne illness and provision for public safety.

Among the advantages for such a reorganization are:

(1) It could designate a specific organization responsible for control of outbreaks. The present system permits the passing of responsibility to other jurisdictions.
(2) It could establish a better system of budgetary control. Money designated for an activity would be used for that specific purpose.
(3) It could implement the recommendations and suggestions made for improving inspectional services without seeking the approval of people from other disciplines who might lack the knowledge for making a correct judgment.
(4) It could establish a system whereby the level of the sanitation of the industry inspected could be assessed and could formulate the inspection program based on that assessment.
(5) It would reduce the cost of inspections by reducing their hidden pyramid cost.
(6) It would centralize the responsibility of recall activities when such action is instituted.

TRAINING PROGRAM FOR FOOD SERVICE PERSONNEL

It should be kept in mind that food that is wholesome when produced or processed may become contaminated with disease-causing agents when improperly handled or prepared for service by personnel not trained in matters of sanitation. This is especially true if their habits of personal hygiene are of a questionable nature. It is therefore important that employees of food-service establishments be given training in the sanitary handling of foods. Such training courses are made available by a number of state and local departments of health. During its 1979 meeting, the Governing Council of the American Public Health Association urged an intensification of such education programs.

Through the efforts of the New York City Board of Health, a course in food sanitation for supervisors and persons in charge of food preparation and service is now required by law in New York City (N.Y. City Health Code 1975). Food handlers must attend the course within 6 months after their employment and must successfully complete it to retain their job.

Karla Longree of the Department of Institution Management, New York State College of Home Economics, Cornell University, in her book *Quality Food Sanitation* (1968), recommends that the subject matter in a sanitation training course include the following:

(1) Elements of microbiology, with emphasis on microorganisms which are important from a public health point of view: Size, shape, spores, reproduction; time-temperature relationships of growth and death; and importance of food as medium for bacteria.
(2) Principles of food preservation.
(3) Parasites in foods.
(4) Transmission of pathogens.
(5) Foodborne illness: Causative organisms, circumstances associated with outbreaks, symptoms; reporting; and the role of the health authority.
(6) Reservoirs of microorganisms: Man (the food handler, the customer); animals (livestock, pets, rodents, insects); environment (sewage, soil, air, water); and food supply.
(7) Contamination of food in the food service area from above reservoirs and from secondary sources such as soiled hands, soiled equipment, utensils, and an ill-maintained physical plant. Control measures: Personal hygiene; rodent and insect control; efficient plumbing; potable water; removal of soil; avoidance of cross-contamination from raw to cooked food; equipment and utensils sanitation; housekeeping in the areas of storage, food preparation, and service.
(8) Multiplication of bacteria in foods and factors affecting multiplication. The meaning of "potentially hazardous foods." Time-temperature relationships; the meaning of "danger zone." Control measures: Time-temperature control for all potentially hazardous foods at all stages of storage, preparation, and service.

Sanitarians who serve as instructors in food sanitation programs may avail themselves of a number of manuals that may act as guidelines. Such manuals are available from the U.S. Department of Health, Education and Welfare, Public Health Service, and Departments of Public Health of various states, municipalities, and countries. Several examples are given below.

U.S. Department of Health, Education and Welfare, Office of Education. *Supervised Food Service Worker. A Suggested Training Program*. Course Unit II (Safe Food Handling, Essential Health Practices, and Sanitation); Course Unit V (Adequate Storage of Food); Teaching the Course. Superintendent of Documents, Washington, D.C. (price 20 cents)

Federal Security Agency, U.S. Public Health Service. From Hand to Mouth. Community Health Series 3. Superintendent of Documents, Washington, D.C. (price 20 cents)

U.S. Department of Health, Education and Welfare, Department of Army, Navy and the Air Force. Sanitary Food Service Instructor's Guide. Public Health Publ. 90. Superintendent of Documents, Washington, D.C.

Edwin Ludewig. New York City Department of Health. Food Sanitation Course, Lecture Notes. 125 Worth Street, New York. (price 60 cents)

New York State Department of Health. Guide for Food Handler Training Course. Flipchart. N.Y. State Dep. of Health, Albany.

Iowa State Department of Health. Sanitation of Food Service Establishments. A Guide for On-the-Job Training of Personnel. Iowa State Dep. of Health, Des Moines.

Washington State Department of Health. Food and Beverage Service Worker's Manual. Wash. State Dep. of Health, Seattle.

Visual aids, such as films, slides, and posters may be obtained from the film libraries of federal and state health agencies and from commercial sources. The U.S. Public Health Service has a film catalog (Publication 776, U.S.P.H.S.) that may be secured from the Superintendent of Documents, Washington, D.C. Films may also be obtained from the Communicable Disease Center, Audiovisual Facility, Atlanta, Georgia. Many films may be borrowed without charge while a rental fee may have to be paid for others.

REFERENCES

BANWART, G.J. 1979. Basic Food Microbiology AVI Publishing Co., Westport, Conn.

GUTHRIE, R.K. 1972. Food Sanitation. AVI Publishing Co., Westport, Conn.

LONGREE, K. 1968. Quality Food Sanitation. Interscience Publishers Division, John Wiley & Sons, New York.

LUKOWSKI, R.F. and ESHBACH, C.E. 1963. Employee Training in Food Service Establishments. Univ. Mass. Coll. Agric., Coop. Ext. Serv., Food Manage. Program Leafl. 7, GPC 3/63 AMA.

N.Y. CITY HEALTH CODE. 1975. Training of Food Sanitarians. N.Y. City Health Code Sect. *87.07.* New York.

N.Y. STATE SANITARY CODE. 1975. Service Food Establishments, Chapter 1, Part 14. N.Y. State Dep. Health, Albany, N.Y. (Section references: 14.10, 14.12, 14.20, 14.40, 14.41, 14.42, 14.46)

U.S. DEP. COMMER. 1979. Food Safety Policy, Scientific and Societal Consideration, Part 2. U.S. Dep. Commer., Natl. Tech. Inf. Serv., Natl. Res. Counc., Washington, D.C.

U.S. DEP. HEALTH, EDUC. WELFARE. 1971. Workshop 3—Prevention of mishandling of foods in commercial and institutional food service operations. *In* Proc. 1971 Natl. Conf. Food Protection, Denver, 1971. U.S. Dep. Health, Educ. Welfare, U.S. Govt. Printing Off., Washington, D.C.

U.S. DEP. HEALTH, EDUC. WELFARE, PUBLIC HEALTH SERV., CENT. DIS. CONTROL. 1978. Foodborne and Waterborne Disease Outbreaks, Annual Survey, 1977. Center for Disease Control, Atlanta.

U.S. DEP. HEALTH, EDUC. WELFARE, PUBLIC HEALTH SERV. 1958. Epidemiology and Control of Foodborne Disease. U.S. Govt. Printing Office, Washington, D.C.

U.S. DEP. HEALTH, EDUC. WELFARE, PUBLIC HEALTH SERV., FOOD DRUG ADMIN. 1976. Food Service Sanitation Manual. U.S. Dep. Health, Educ. Welfare (FDA) *78-2081.* U.S. Govt. Printing Off., Washington, D.C.

26

Investigation of Foodborne Disease Outbreaks

When a disease is common to or affecting a large number of persons in a community in a short period of time, it is said to be epidemic. If the cases are limited to a specific group of individuals, such as a family, a group partaking of a home-prepared meal, or persons eating at a public establishment or at a banquet, the occurrence may then be considered to be an outbreak rather than an epidemic.

As previously stated, any raw foods previous to cooking may contain microorganisms capable of causing gastroenteritis. Most foods, if improperly cooked, prepared, stored, or refrigerated, are subject to contamination with pathogenic microorganisms. This is especially true of foods that can support bacterial multiplication and the production of enterotoxins. Some foods may inadvertently be tainted with inorganic toxic chemicals.

Reports of investigations of several such outbreaks have been included in the text to serve as illustrations of the practical application of the epidemiologic information given regarding the toxic agents associated with foodborne diseases.

Public health officials are charged with the investigation of outbreaks of gastroenteritis. The aim of these investigations is: (1) to determine the cause of the outbreak, (2) to find the item of food responsible for the illness, (3) to take steps to arrest further spread of the outbreak, and (4) to educate responsible individuals in the prevention of similar occurrences. It is hoped that this outline may serve as an aid to public health workers and others engaged in such investigations. It is regrettable that only the fundamentals pertaining to these investigations can be given since foodborne outbreaks differ in their characteristics, requiring the investigator to use judgment in his undertaking. With experience he will become more proficient in carrying out the aims enumerated. It is suggested that, whenever possible, individuals who intend to engage in such investigations be prepared by having previously familiarized themselves with the following knowledge:

(1) Various types of foodborne infections
(2) Epidemiological characteristics of such outbreaks
(3) Clinical symptoms of resulting illness
(4) Knowledge of food sanitation
(5) Foods most vulnerable to bacterial contamination
(6) Laboratory tests available to determine causative agents

CAUSATIVE AGENTS OF FOODBORNE DISEASE

(1) Bacteria and their enterotoxins
(2) Viruses
(3) Protozoans
(4) Helminths (intestinal worms)
(5) Poisonous fungi
(6) Toxic chemicals
(7) Poisonous plants
(8) Toxic animal products

INVESTIGATION OF OUTBREAKS

(1) Report outbreak to local or state health department
(2) Prompt action when outbreak is reported
(3) Visit homes of persons involved (the ill as well as those not made ill)
(4) Interview as many persons as possible who partook of the food
(5) Obtain specimens of stool and/or vomitus from ill persons
(6) Visit establishment where food was prepared, served, and eaten, and secure menu of foods served
(7) Interview food handlers
(8) Obtain samples of suspected foods
(9) Make a sanitary inspection of food handling establishment
(10) Arrange for the laboratory examination of food samples and specimens

INTERVIEWING OF INVOLVED PERSONS

Persons who become ill, as well as those who remained well, should be interviewed. The latter serve as the control group in your search for the food item responsible for the outbreak.

Prepare a questionnaire suitable for the outbreak to be completed for each person. It should contain pertinent questions, such as:

(1) Did you become ill?
(2) If so, how soon after eating did illness occur?
(3) What symptoms did you have?
(4) How long did illness last?
(5) What is the name of the physician who attended you?
(6) What foods on the menu did you eat?
(7) Did appearance, taste, or odor of any items of food appear unusual?

In interviewing the food handlers, the following should be obtained:

(1) If home outbreak, name, place, and date of purchase of food
(2) How it was prepared, stored, and refrigerated
(3) Examine hands and face of food handler for open lesions
(4) Inquire regarding recent illnesses of food handler, such as: gastroenteritis, common cold, sore throat, and jaundice
(5) Determine whether any toxic metal kitchen utensils are used
(6) Are cleaning agents, pesticides, or lye kept in areas where food is prepared?
(7) Look for evidence of roach or rat infestation

ANALYSIS OF INFORMATION COLLECTED

Prepare a master chart from the information in the questionnaires. Tabulate all the available information. Determine from the master chart the mean incubation period of the outbreak. This is helpful in forming a hypothesis as to what the causative agent may be. For example, if it is found that the incubation period was less than 1 hr, a metallic poison or a toxic alkaloid should be suspected; if it was 2 to 6 hr, a staphylococcal intoxication may be involved; if 8 hr or more, then an enteric infection can be expected, such as salmonellosis.

Determine the attack rate of each food item on the menu eaten by those made ill and those who remained well. The food item with a significantly increased attack rate among the ill persons as compared with the rate among those who were not ill may be considered to be the food responsible for acting as the vehicle of transmission of the infective agent. The determination of attack rates of foods involved in foodborne outbreaks under investigation is subsequently described in detail in this chapter when the use of investigatory forms is discussed.

Should the laboratory find the same microorganisms of similar serotype, phage type, or other definite type or toxin in the suspected food as those isolated from specimens of vomitus or feces submitted by the sick patients, then the investigation has been productive, and the vehicle of transmission as well as the etiologic agent responsible for the outbreak has been definitely determined.

FOLLOW-UP

Revisit establishment where the food was served and eaten. Placing emphasis on the incriminated food, obtain details on: (1) its source, (2) date of purchase, (3) method of preparation, (4) date of preparation, (5) its storage previous to cooking, and (6) pay special attention to its refrigeration before and after cooking.

If indicated, visit retailer or wholesaler where food was purchased and take whatever action you feel is necessary to prevent further spread of infection. If the dealers are outside your jurisdiction, notify the state department for follow-up.

CONTROL MEASURES AND PREVENTION

Food handlers should be educated regarding proper sanitary measures in food preparation, with emphasis placed on thorough cooking of all foods, prompt refrigeration of all perishable foods, exclusion from food handling of all persons with pyogenic skin infections, gastrointestinal symptoms, or upper respiratory infection.

Should botulism be suspected, appropriate type of specific (or bivalent or trivalent) antitoxin should be administered within 36 hr to all persons who have eaten the incriminated food. An immediate search must be made for all such persons. If canned food is involved, it should be embargoed, samples for laboratory study be taken, and prompt notification of the Food and Drug Administration be made.

INVESTIGATORY FORMS

As an aid to public health personnel engaged in the investigation of food-related illness, the Committee on Communicable Diseases Affecting Man, International Association of Milk, Food, and Environmental Sanitation, Ames, Iowa, has prepared a series of forms to be used in such investigations. Their use makes for a complete investigation of such illness whether it occurs endemically or in the form of an outbreak. Completion of the forms should result in a successful undertaking. The forms are available from the association in tablet pads of 100. With the permission of the association, copies of the forms are given in this chapter.

Form A

When a report of illness attributed to food is initially received, usually by telephone, information may be recorded on Form A (Food-Related Alert/Complaint Record). The complainant should be questioned as to the time of onset of the first symptoms of illness, the number and location of persons known to have become ill, the name of the food suspected to have caused the illness, and the place at which the stricken person(s) ate the food. The complainant should be asked to retain all suspected foods and their containers. He should be instructed on how to collect specimens of vomitus and/or feces samples from all sick persons and to refrigerate them until they are picked up by the investigator.

The investigation should be started promptly while the memory of foods eaten by the affected persons is still fresh. The early identification of the offending article of food may prevent additional illness by stopping its further distribution and sale, and by recalling lots that have already been distributed.

Form B

When interviewing as many involved individuals as possible by personal visit or by telephone, Form B (Case History) should be completed for each ill person as well as for those who remained well. Clinical data regarding their illness and information pertaining to the foods eaten is thus obtained.

Form C

After it has been determined from the information obtained that the outbreak is really due to foodborne disease, the accumulated data may now be entered on Form C (Summary of Case Histories). As most persons will give more or less similar information, the form may be used initially in most routine outbreaks. A graph or curve may be plotted depicting the distribution of the initial symptoms of the cases. Such a graph, if it is characterized by a sharp rise of cases to a peak with a gradual fall as the outbreak progresses, will help determine whether the outbreak originated from a common source (Fig. 26.1). It is important at this time to notify the district or state epidemiologist regarding the outbreak.

Form D

Clinical specimens of vomitus, fecal samples, rectal swabs, and blood specimens for agglutination tests should be obtained as soon as possible

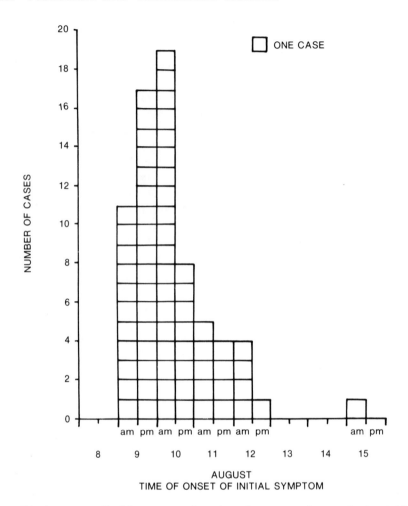

Numbers on vertical line represent number of cases; numbers on horizontal line represent days of the month or hours of the day, each block represents one case.

Courtesy of International Assoc. of Milk Food, and Environmental Sanitarians

FIG. 26.1. COMMON SOURCE EPIDEMIOLOGIC CURVE

after the onset of illness in appropriate sterile containers. Form D (Clinical Specimen Collection Report) should be made out for each specimen and a copy accompany each sample to the laboratory. When the laboratory reports are received, copies should be sent to the patients' physicians.

FOOD-RELATED ALERT/COMPLAINT RECORD

Form A

Complaint Received From	Address	Phone
Person to Contact for More Information	Address	Phone: Home Work

Complaint

Illness ☐ Yes[1,2] ☐ No	Number Ill	Time Illness Began Date Hour	Predominant Symptoms		
Suspect Foods[3]		Source	Brand Identification		Lot Number
Suspect Meals		Place	Address		
Persons Attending Suspect Meal			Address		Phone

Places Foods Eaten (last 72 hours)	Date	Time	Address
Today			
Yesterday			
Day before yesterday			

Received By	Date	Time

Action Taken	Nature of Complaint:
	☐ Illness ☐ Unsanitary Establishment ☐ Contaminated, Adulterated Spoiled Food ☐ Other (Specify)

[1] If yes, professional staff member should obtain information about patient and record on Form B.
[2] Ask person to collect vomitus or stool in a clean jar; wrap, identify, and refrigerate; hold until health official makes further arrangements.
[3] Ask person to refrigerate all food eaten during the 72 hours before onset of illness; save or retrieve original containers or packages; sample should be properly identified; hold until health official makes further arrangements.

Courtesy of International Assoc. of Milk, Food, and Environmental Sanitarians

FIG. 26.2. INVESTIGATORY FORM A

CASE HISTORY: CLINICAL DATA

Form B—Part 1 of 2 Parts

Name		Place of Outbreak, if known	Complaint Number	Identification Number

| | | Address | | Phone: Home Work |

| Age | Sex | Special dietary habits, Ethnic group, or other personal data | Occupation | Place of work |

Signs and Symptoms:† (Check appropriate signs and symptoms and circle those that occurred first)

INTOXICATIONS
- *☐ Nausea
- *☐ Vomiting
- ☐ Bloating
- ☐ Burning sensation (mouth)
- ☐ Cyanosis
- ☐ Excessive salivation
- ☐ Flushing
- ☐ Itching
- ☐ Metallic taste
- ☐ Prostration
- ☐ Thirst
- ☐ Others (specify)

ENTERIC INFECTIONS
- *☐ Abdominal cramps
- *☐ Diarrhea
  - ☐ Bloody
  - ☐ Mucoid
  - ☐ Watery
  - ☐ No./day ____
- *☐ Fever
  - Degrees ____ F ____ C
  - ☐ Chills
  - ☐ Constipation

GENERALIZED INFECTIONS
- ☐ Cough
- ☐ Dehydration
- ☐ Edema
- ☐ Headache
- ☐ Jaundice
- ☐ Lack of appetite
- ☐ Myalgia
- ☐ Perspiration
- ☐ Rash
- ☐ Weakness

NEUROLOGICAL ILLNESSES
- ☐ Blurred vision
- ☐ Coma
- ☐ Delirium
- ☐ Difficulty in Speaking
- ☐ Difficulty in Swallowing
- ☐ Dizziness
- ☐ Double vision
- ☐ Numbness
- ☐ Paralysis
- ☐ Pupils: ☐ dilated, ☐ fixed, or ☐ constricted
- ☐ Tingling

Time of Onset: Date Hour	Time of Eating Suspect Food or Meal Date Hour	Place of Eating Suspect Food or Meal	Fatal: ☐ Yes ☐ No	Incubation Period	Duration of Illness

Medications Taken for Illness	Known Allergies	Medications/Inoculations Taken Before Illness		

Physician Consulted	Address	Phone	Hospital Attended	Address

Contacts with Known Cases Before Illness (Names)	Address		Phone

Cases in Household Occurring Subsequently (Names)		Dates of Onset

Type of Specimens Obtained	Date Collected	Identification Number	Laboratory Results
1.			
2.			
3.			

†Signs and symptoms are listed in columns to suggest classification of the disease; their occurrence is not necessarily limited to the category in which they appear on this form.
*Ask if these symptoms occurred, even if they were not mentioned in the interview.

(See reverse side)

Courtesy of International Assoc. of Milk, Food, and Environmental Sanitarians

FIG. 26.3. INVESTIGATORY FORM B. PART 1

CASE HISTORY: FOOD HISTORY AND COMMON SOURCES

Form B—Part 2 of 2 Parts

☐ Ill
☐ Well

Day of Illness/Outbreak. Date _____

Breakfast[2] _____ Hour _____

Place _____
Items[3] _____

Lunch[2] _____ Hour _____

Place _____

Dinner[2] _____ Hour _____

Place _____

Snacks[2] _____ Hour _____

Source _____

Day Before Illness/Outbreak. Date _____

Breakfast[2] _____ Hour _____

Place _____

Lunch[2] _____ Hour _____

Place _____

Dinner[2] _____ Hour _____

Place _____

Snacks[2] _____ Hour _____

Source _____

Two Days Before Illness. Date _____

Breakfast[2] _____ Hour _____

Place _____

Lunch[2] _____ Hour _____

Place _____

Dinner[2] _____ Hour _____

Place _____

Snacks[2] _____ Hour _____

Source _____

History of Eating Suspicious Food Earlier Than 2 Days Before Illness:

Item	Date of Eating	Source	Address

General Information:

Common Events or Gatherings	Date	Persons Attending	Address	Phone

Nonroutine Travel (locations)

Water supply[3]	Sewage Disposal[3]	Pet/Animals (Kind and Number of Each)

Remarks

Investigator	Title	Agency	Date

[1]Include all foods, ice, and beverages.
[2]Record names of persons eating same meal and whether or not ill.
[3]Specify m for municipal or p for private and type of private installation.

INVESTIGATORY FORM B. PART 2

SUMMARY OF CASE HISTORIES

Form C—Part 1 of 2 Parts

ID No.	Name of Ill Person or Well Person (List all exposed persons whether or not ill)	Address	Phone	Sex	Age	Time of Eating		Time of Initial Symptom		Incubation Period (Difference Between Eating and Onset)	Signs and Symptoms										Severity			
						Day	Hour	Day	Hour		Nausea	Vomiting	Abdominal cramps	Diarrhea	Fever					Duration	Physician Seen	Hospitalized	Death

Place of Outbreak _____ Dates of Outbreak _____ Complaint Number _____

Investigator _____ Title _____   Median _____ Suspected Etiology _____

Fold here   (See reverse side)

Courtesy of International Assoc. of Milk, Food, and Environmental Sanitarians

FIG. 26.4. INVESTIGATORY FORM C. PART 1

SUMMARY OF CASE HISTORIES

Form C—Part 2 of 2 Parts

NOTE: Line-up with appropriate identification number of Part 1-Form C

Foods Eaten

Laboratory Tests

Specimen

Date

Organism

Specific comments or additional information about any ill/not ill persons (Record all information where space does not permit in other sections, such as additional symptoms, physician, and hospital names)

ID No.

Suspect Food

Confirmed Etiology

Remarks

· Fold here

INVESTIGATORY FORM C. PART 2

CLINICAL SPECIMEN COLLECTION REPORT

	Complaint Number	Specimen Number

Form D

Place of Outbreak	Address	ID Number	Type of Specimen

Person from whom Specimen Obtained	Address	Phone

Reason for Collecting Specimen:
☐ Victim of outbreak, ☐ Person at risk but not ill, ☐ Handler of suspect food, ☐ Suspected carrier, ☐ Animal, ☐ Other (specify) _____

Physician	Address	Phone

Symptoms:
☐ Nausea, ☐ Vomiting, ☐ Abdominal cramps, ☐ Diarrhea, ☐ Fever, ☐ Others (specify) _____

Time of Eating: Day Hour	Time of Onset: Day Hour	Incubation Period	Duration of Illness
Method of Collecting Specimens		Method of Preservation	Method of Shipment

Other Information

Investigator Collecting Specimen	Title	Agency	Date/Hour: Collected Submitted

Tests Requested:	Presence/ Absence	Count	Definitive Type
☐ Staphylococci			
☐ Beta Hemolytic Streptococci			
☐ C. perfringens			
☐ Salmonella			
☐ Shigella			
☐ E. coli			
☐ V. parahaemolyticus			
☐ Botulinus toxin			
☐ Others (specify)			

Comments and Interpretations

Laboratory Analyst	Agency	Date/Hour: Received	Started	Completed	Etiologic Agent

Courtesy of International Assoc. of Milk, Food and Environmental Sanitarians

FIG. 26.5. INVESTIGATORY FORM D

Form E

Each sample of food, when available, should be collected aseptically and sent to the laboratory with a completed copy of Form E (Food/Environmental Sample Collection Report).

From the presently attainable evidence, it may be possible for the investigator to make a hypothesis regarding the probable food responsible for the illness, the infective agent, and the source of infection. Further study on his part will determine whether or not his assumptions are substantiated.

Form F

It is now important for the investigator to visit the location where the suspected food was produced, processed, prepared, stored, or served. He should be accompanied by a trained sanitarian so that while he is obtaining epidemiologic information, questioning, and examining the food handlers for illness or skin lesions, and securing from the workers whatever laboratory specimens are indicated, the sanitarian can do a thorough sanitary inspection of the premises and the kitchen, inquire into the processing and preparation of foods, check storage facilities, refrigeration temperatures, dishwashing equipment, garbage disposal methods, look for evidence of cooked foods in contact with raw foods, rodent infestation, and other sanitary violations. The sanitarian may employ Form F (Food Preparation Review) to enter his findings.

It is helpful in determining the causative agent to find the mean or median incubation period of the outbreak. The latter is preferable and is obtained by locating the mid-value of a listing of the incubation periods of all the cases in a series from the shortest to the longest period. If the series consists of an even number of values, the average of the 2 middle values would be the median.

Form G

The next step is to calculate from the collected data the food-specific attack rate of each item of food on the menu by completing Form G (Food-Specific Attack Rate Table). Thus a comparison is made of the percentage of ill persons who ate each food with the percentage of ill persons who did not eat each food. It will be found that the food responsible for the illness will usually have the highest attack rate in the column for persons who ate the food and the lowest attack rate in the column for persons who did not eat the food. The difference between these 2 rates will be the greatest.

FOOD/ENVIRONMENTAL SAMPLE COLLECTION REPORT

	Complaint Number	Sample Number[1]

Form E

Place Collected	Address		Phone

Person-In-Charge	Sample		Date/Hour Collected

Reason for Collecting Sample:
☐ Food from alleged outbreak,   ☐ Food ingredient,   ☐ Similar food prepared in similar manner to that involved in outbreak,
☐ Special survey,   ☐ Routine,   ☐ Environmental,   ☐ Other (specify) _____

Method of Collecting and Shipping Sample:
Method of Sterilizing: Container[2] | Collection Utensil[2]

Location Food Stored When Sampled	Temperature: Food	Storage Unit	Time Between Serving and Sampling

Shipped: ☐ Refrigerated, ☐ Frozen, ☐ Ambient	Identification Marks	Cost of Sample

Product Identification: Name	Brand	Lot Number

Manufacturer's Name	Address	Container Size or Weight

Symptoms of Victims:
☐ Nausea,   ☐ Vomiting,   ☐ Abdominal Cramps,   ☐ Fever,   ☐ Diarrhea   ☐ Other (specify) _____

Time of Eating Suspect Food/Meal: Date Hour	Time of Onset: Date Hour	Incubation Period	Duration of Illness

Investigator	Title	Agency	Date

Test Requested	Presence/ Absence	Count/Concentration	Definitive Type
☐ Staphylococci			
☐ Staphyloenterotoxin			
☐ C. perfringens			
☐ B. cereus			
☐ Salmonella			
☐ Shigella			
☐ E. coli			
☐ V. parahaemolyticus			
☐ C. botulinum			
☐ Botulinus toxin			
☐ Chemical			
☐ Aerobic Colony Count			
☐ Coliform			
☐ Enterococci			
☐ Other (specify)			

Condition of Food	pH	a_w	Temperature: When received

Comments and interpretations

Laboratory Analyst	Agency	Date/Hour: Received	Started	Completed	Agent Identified

[1] Attach a list of number, sample, and tests desired for other samples collected at the same establishment during the same investigation.
[2] Specify only if unusual (such as field) method of sterilizing or sanitizing collection container or utensil or collecting sample is used.

Courtesy of International Assoc. of Milk, Food, and Environmental Sanitarians

FIG. 26.6. INVESTIGATORY FORM E

TABLE 26.1. FOOD SPECIFIC ATTACK RATE

Foods	Number of Persons Who Ate Specific Foods				Number of Persons Who Did Not Eat Specific Foods				Difference in %
	Ill	Not Ill	Total	% Ill	Ill	Not Ill	Total	% Ill	
Braised beef	74	17	91	81	2	9	11	18	+63
Peas	48	20	68	71	28	6	34	82	−11
Cabbage salad	36	12	48	75	40	14	54	74	+ 1
Buttered biscuits	46	12	58	79	30	14	44	68	+11
Peaches	62	22	84	73	14	4	18	78	− 5
Milk	60	16	76	79	16	10	26	62	+17

Source: Anon (1975).

In Table 26.1, the attack rate for persons who ate braised beef (the offending food in the cited outbreak) was 81%, while the attack rate for persons who did not eat braised beef was only 18%. The difference between the 2 percentages was +63, indicating that braised beef was the suspect food. The 2 persons who became ill, although they said they had not eaten the incriminated food, either forgot what they had eaten, or their delicate makeup caused sympathetic vomiting or other symptoms. On the other hand, the 9 individuals who ate the alleged contaminated food and did not become ill were either more resistant to gastrointestinal infection than the average person, or, because of the usual uneven distribution of the infective agent in the food, they may have received a portion free of contaminant.

Form H

The combination of the clinical symptoms, the epidemiologic findings, and the laboratory reports will now confirm or refute the original hypothesis as to the agent responsible for the outbreak of illness. The sanitary report as to how the food in question was processed, prepared, and handled should reveal the point at which contamination occurred. It will now be possible to prepare a report of the outbreak. It may be written in a narrative form as the illustration of the various investigations made by the author, or Form H (Foodborne Illness Summary Report) may be used. When completed, Form H should contain all the pertinent information pertaining to the outbreak. A copy of the report should be submitted to the agency, state or federal, that is responsible for foodborne disease surveillance.

The identification of a contaminated or otherwise hazardous food product and its removal from the market will prevent further illness from the same source. The correction of any faulty condition found to have been

FOOD PREPARATION REVIEW

Form F—Part 1 of 2 Parts

				Complaint Number
Establishment: (Name)	Address			Phone
Person-in-charge	Type of Establishment	Date of Outbreak	Date and Time of Suspected Meal	
Suspect Food:	Source	Address		Date Received
Brand	Container Size or Weight	Manufacturer's Name	Address	Lot Number

Ingredients	Sources

Operational Step	Method	Type of Equipment	Temperature	Time	Names of Workers Involved	Remarks (History of Illness or Infection of Workers, Sanitation Unusual Events, Other Information)

Interpretation	Height ______; Length ______ and Width ______; or Diameter ______ of Storage Pot, Pan, or Container

(See reverse side)

Courtesy of International Assoc. of Milk, Food and Environmental Sanitarians

FIG. 26.7. INVESTIGATORY FORM F. PART 1

FOOD PREPARATION REVIEW FORM

Form F—Part 2 of 2 Parts

Food	Method of Processing or Preparing Food Used (e.g. frozen, canned, baked)

Operational Procedures Contributing to Outbreak (One or more should be checked):

☐ Inadequate refrigeration. ☐ Inadequate hot holding. ☐ Preparing foods several hours before serving. ☐ Anaerobic packaging. ☐ Inadequate cooking. ☐ Inadequate reheating.
☐ Obtaining foods from unsafe sources, ☐ Using contaminated raw ingredients in uncooked product. ☐ Food contaminated by infected person. ☐ Cross-contamination.
☐ Inadequate cleaning of equipment. ☐ Poor dry storage practices, ☐ Toxic container. ☐ Addition of poisonous chemical. ☐ Natural toxicant in plant or animal by raw food.
☐ Other (specify) _____

Description of Operations and Deficiencies:

Control Action Taken:

Investigator	Title	Agency	Date of Investigation

Laboratory Results:

Food and Environment

Sample or Swab	Sample No.	Organism/Toxin	Count	Specimen	Specimen No.	Organism and Definitive Type

Workers

Interpretation and Remarks

Laboratory Analyst	Agency	Date: Received	Started	Completed	Etiologic Agent	Source of Contamination

INVESTIGATORY FORM F. PART 2

FOOD-SPECIFIC ATTACK RATE TABLE

Form G

| | | Place of Outbreak | | | | | Complaint Number |

Food	Number of Persons Who Ate Specific Food			Number of Persons Who Did Not Eat Specific Food			Difference In Percent	Significance
	Ill	Well	Total	Percent Ill	Ill	Well	Total	Percent Ill

Remarks and Interpretation

Suspect Food

Courtesy of International Assoc. of Milk, Food, and Environmental Sanitarians

FIG. 26.8. INVESTIGATORY FORM G

FOODBORNE ILLNESS SUMMARY REPORT Form H	Complaint Number	Agent and Definitive Type	Disease
Location: City	County		State/Province

Date of Onset of First Case	Number Ill	Number at Risk	Number Hospitalized	Fatalities

Symptom (Percentage):

Nausea _____,   Vomiting _____,   Abdominal Cramps _____,   Diarrhea _____,

Fever _____,   Other (specify) _____

Duration of Illness (Hours):   Shortest _____,   Longest _____,   Median _____

Incubation Period:

Shortest _____

Longest _____

Median _____

Responsible Vehicle (Food)	Method of Processing or Preparing Food

Place Foods Eaten (Check one):
- ☐ Food Service Establishment
- ☐ School
- ☐ Medical care facility
- ☐ Other institution (Type _____)
- ☐ Home
- ☐ Camp
- ☐ Picnic
- ☐ Intransit Carriers (Type _____)
- ☐ Others (specify) _____
  _____

Place Food Contaminated or Mishandled

(Check one, occasionally more)[1]:
- ☐ Farm
- ☐ Stream or bay, etc. (Name _____)
- ☐ Processing Plant
  - ☐ Milk
  - ☐ Bakery
  - ☐ Canning
  - ☐ Frozen food
  - ☐ Meat
  - ☐ Poultry
  - ☐ Fish
  - ☐ Egg
  - ☐ Other (Type _____)
- ☐ Warehouse or storage
- ☐ Transportation (Type _____)
- ☐ Vending machine
- ☐ Retail store
- ☐ Home
- ☐ Food service establishment
  - ☐ Table service
  - ☐ Cafeteria
  - ☐ Fast food service
  - ☐ Take out
  - ☐ Banquet
  - ☐ Smorgasbord
  - ☐ Catering
  - ☐ Mobile/itinerant
  - ☐ Delicatessen
  - ☐ Tavern or bar
  - ☐ Other _____
- ☐ Other (specify) _____

Factors Contributing to Outbreak (Check all appropriate):
- ☐ Inadequate refrigeration
- ☐ Inadequate hot holding
- ☐ Preparing foods several hours before serving
- ☐ Anaerobic packaging
- ☐ Inadequate cooking or thermal processing
- ☐ Inadequate reheating
- ☐ Obtaining foods from unsafe sources
- ☐ Using contaminated raw ingredients in uncooked product
- ☐ Food contaminated by infected person
- ☐ Cross contaminated by raw foods
- ☐ Inadequate cleaning of equipment
- ☐ Poor dry storage practices
- ☐ Toxic container
- ☐ Addition of poisonous chemical
- ☐ Natural toxicant in plant or animal
- ☐ Other (specify) _____
  _____

Agent Isolated From (Check All Appropriate)

Count/Type
- ☐ Persons ill (Number ___)   _____
- ☐ Responsible vehicle   _____
- ☐ Worker(s) (Number ___)   _____
- ☐ Raw food   _____
- ☐ Ingredient (Type _____)   _____
- ☐ Equipment (Type _____)   _____
- ☐ Environment (specify _____
  _____)   _____
- ☐ Other (specify _____
  _____)   _____

Attachments with Report:
- ☐ Summary of case histories (Part 2)[2]
- ☐ Epidemic curve
- ☐ Laboratory reports (specimens)
- ☐ Laboratory reports (samples)
- ☐ Food-specific attack rate table[2]
- ☐ Food preparation review[2]
- ☐ Narrative (may be put on reverse side)
- ☐ Recommendations for prevention
- ☐ Other (specify) _____
  _____

Investigator	Reporting Agency	Date

[1]If more than one checked, signify c for contamination; m for mishandling before box.

[2]These should always be attached.

Courtesy of International Assoc. of Milk, Food, and Environmental Sanitarians

FIG. 26.9. INVESTIGATORY FORM H

responsible for the outbreak should be called to the attention of managers, employees, and homemakers so that repetition of similar unwholesome conditions may be avoided in the future.

NOTE

The epidemiologist, while conducting an investigation of a food-related outbreak, cannot determine beyond question the etiologic agent responsible for the series of illnesses. He can decide by epidemiologic means what was the vehicle of transmission or the item(s) of food involved, but he can only predicate which microorganisms or what toxic product is the causative agent. It is necessary for him to solicit the assistance of the laboratory for that determination. Samples of available food and specimens from patients must be examined before it may be said that the investigation has been satisfactorily completed.

Readers interested in laboratory procedures relating to food microbiology are referred to the *Compendium of Methods for the Microbiological Evaluation of Foods*, edited by M.L. Speck (1976) and published by the American Public Health Association, Washington, D.C.

REFERENCES

ANON. 1975. Procedures to Investigate Foodborne Illness, 3rd Edition. Intern. Assoc. of Milk, Food, and Environmental Sanitation. P.O. Box 701, Ames, Iowa 50010.

BRYAN, F.L. 1974. Bacteriological food hazards today—based on epidemiological information. Food Technol. *28* (9) 57.

DACK, G.M. 1956. Food Poisoning, 3rd Edition. Univ. of Chicago Press, Chicago.

GUTHRIE, R.K. 1972. Food Sanitation. AVI Publishing Co., Westport, Conn.

PHILLIPS, S.F. 1975. Diarrhea. Pathogenesis and diagnostic techniques. Postgrad. Med. *57*, 65.

SPECK, M.L. 1976. Compendium of Methods for the Microbiological Evaluation of Foods. American Public Health Association, Washington, D.C.

THATCHER, F.S. and CLARK, D.S. 1968. Microorganisms in Foods. Their Significances and Methods of Enumeration. Univ. of Toronto Press, Toronto.

U.S. DEP. HEALTH, EDUC. WELFARE, PUBLIC HEALTH SERV., FOOD DRUG ADMIN. 1976. Food Service Sanitation Manual. Dep. Health, Educ. Welfare (FDA) *78–2081*.

WEISER, H.H., MOUNTNEY, G.J. and GOULD, W.A. 1971. Practical Food Microbiology and Technology, 2nd Edition. AVI Publishing Co., Westport, Conn.

27

Gastrointestinal Illness Aboard Cruise Ships and Aircraft

The occurrence of typhoid fever among passengers of a cruise ship on the St. Lawrence River is described in Chapter 3. As food and water are consumed by passengers on cruise ships and aircraft, the risk of gastrointestinal illness among such persons is possible unless the source of the food and water is from reliable and approved sources and strict sanitary handling is maintained by those responsible for the preparation and service of the food. It is also of utmost importance that the potability of water be maintained aboard the vessel and that water from questionable sources be avoided.

Public health officials are urged to report cases of gastrointestinal illness that may have been acquired aboard cruise ships and aircraft to the Enteric Disease Branch, Bacterial Disease Division, or Quarantine Division, Bureau of Epidemiology, Center for Disease Control.

Certain logistic problems complicate the investigation of outbreaks that occur aboard cruise vessels and aircraft. Passengers may not become ill until after disembarkation. Notification of health authorities frequently occurs after arrival of the ship or plane. Passengers disperse to multiple destinations soon after they disembark, and schedules frequently dictate that planes and ships depart within hours after arrival. Therefore, time to organize and conduct an investigation is frequently very limited. Such investigations require close cooperation among responsible federal, state, and local agencies. Prompt reporting of diarrheal illness aboard aircraft and vessels by the aircraft pilot or vessel master is essential to permit time to plan an investigation.

After such an incident is reported, the need for a full investigation is determined by the severity, timing, and magnitude of the problem. These investigations usually include questionnaire surveys of passengers and crew, detailed evaluation of sanitation, and laboratory analysis of food, water, environmental, and patient specimens. Several such investigations made by the Quarantine Division of the Center for Disease Control are given below.

GASTROINTESTINAL ILLNESS ABOARD CRUISE SHIPS

Salmonellosis

During a cruise aboard a Caribbean cruise ship in 1974, 53 out of 740 passengers came down with severe gastroenteritis. *Salmonella bareilly* was isolated from stool specimens obtained from 15 ill passengers. During the ship's next 6 cruises, 6 different serotypes of *Salmonella* were isolated from fecal specimens of ill passengers, and 10 different serotypes from crew members. Environmental investigation revealed cross-connection between raw and cooked food in the galley and inadequate refrigeration of foods during the breakfast, lunch, and midnight buffets. Control measures consisted of removing culture-positive food handlers from work, separation of raw and cooked foods, and adequate refrigeration of foods served at the buffets.

That same year, another outbreak of salmonellosis occurred involving 118 passengers and crew members aboard another cruise ship that sailed from Miami on a Caribbean 2-week cruise. *Salmonella enteritidis* was isolated from fecal cultures obtained from 50 of 71 ill passengers. None of the food items could be significantly statistically associated with the illness. However, *S. enteritidis* was isolated from the potable water distribution system aboard ship.

Shigellosis

An explosive waterborne outbreak of shigellosis involving approximately 690 passengers and crew aboard a cruise ship in the Caribbean Sea occurred in June 1973. Epidemiologic investigation implicated water and ice aboard the ship as the vehicles of transmission. Water samples obtained from the distribution system contained elevated fecal coliform counts, and cultures indicated the presence of *Shigella*. It was believed that the flushing of a water holding tank with water from a fire hydrant aboard the ship permitted *Shigella* organisms originally present in the salt water in the fire system to enter the potable water tanks.

Vibrio parahaemolyticus Gastroenteritis

During the first 2 months of 1975, large outbreaks of *V. parahaemolyticus* gastroenteritis occurred on 2 cruise ships.

Diarrheal illness was reported among 252 (36%) of 703 passengers aboard a cruise ship, the outbreak peaking on January 2. *V. parahaemolyticus* was isolated from rectal swabs taken on ill passengers and crew members. Cultures were made of foods, beverages, potable water and ice, and environmental surfaces in the ship's galley. A seafood cocktail that consisted of frozen shrimp, canned crabmeat, and frozen grouper, served to the passengers at dinner on January 1, was found to be the vehicle of transmission of the vibrio. Contamination of the cocktail occurred as the cleaning of the shrimp was done on a food preparation surface that had been splashed with the ship's circulating salt water system from which *V. parahaemolyticus* was cultured. Control measures consisted of a review of appropriate food handling practices with the ship's personnel and removal of the salt water outlet in the ship's galley.

A similar outbreak of *V. parahaemolyticus* occurred on the cruise of February 8 to 20 on another cruise ship on which 447 (61%) of 734 passengers and 29 (5%) of 586 crew members experienced diarrheal illness with *V. parahaemolyticus* isolated from rectal swabs from 19 passengers and crew members. Investigation incriminated shrimp cocktail served at dinner of the fifth day and lobster served at dinner on the eleventh day. The incriminated food was precooked and frozen; it thawed at room temperature for approximately 8 hr. While thawing, it was washed with sea water, which is available throughout the ship in the fire system. The shrimp were reportedly washed in salted potable water after cooking and cleaning, so their source of contamination remains unclear. Control measures included termination of use of sea water in food handling areas.

Trichinosis

A retrospective investigation in which passengers were contacted by letter or telephone was made following reports of illness that occurred in persons who had taken a trip aboard a cruise ship between August 24 and September 7, 1974. The ship had sailed round trip from San Francisco to Juneau, stopping at 6 ports of call in Canada and Alaska. The illness was diagnosed as trichinosis and occurred in 13 passengers.

An analysis of the food histories obtained from the ill passengers revealed a statistically significant association between becoming ill and having a preference for chopped beef items that appeared on the menu. As a single meat grinder had been used in the ship galley for both pork and beef products, it led to the speculation that a ground beef preparation may have been inadvertently contaminated with raw pork and may have been served without being adequately cooked. The use of separate meat grinders for beef and pork was recommended.

Coliform Bacilli in Potable Water

Two outbreaks of gastroenteritis occurred in 1976 on the same ship during 2 separate Caribbean cruises. On the first trip 35% of the passengers and on the second voyage 56% were affected. Coliform bacilli were found in the potable water system although ultraviolet light was used to purify the water.

A marked decline in diarrheal outbreaks on cruise vessels is attributed to the cruise vessel sanitary inspection program which has been rigorously administered since 1974. All vessels with a home port in the United States must meet the U.S. Public Health Standards. They are inspected and reinspected until the standards are maintained.

GASTROINTESTINAL ILLNESS ON AIRCRAFT

Staphylococcus Food Poisoning

An outbreak of gastrointestinal illness occurred in October 1973 among economy class passengers on 3 separate flights on the same aircraft that originated in southern Europe. A custard dessert prepared at a catering facility in Lisbon, Portugal, and served to the economy class passengers on each of the flights was incriminated. It was learned that during preparation the custard was held at a temperature of about 15.6°C (60°F) for over 4 hr. *Staphylococcus aureus*, phage nontypical and penicillin resistant, was isolated from samples of custard as well as from specimens of feces from affected passengers.

Gastrointestinal illness occurred among 15 out of 1855 passengers on an American carrier en route from Rio de Janeiro, Brazil, to New York City. Chocolate eclairs consumed aboard the flight were found to be contaminated with type D staphylococcal enterotoxin. The eclairs were prepared in Rio de Janeiro and had been left unrefrigerated for about 10 hr before being placed aboard the aircraft.

On February 2, 1975, a total of 196 (57%) out of 343 passengers and 1 out of 20 crew members aboard a chartered commercial aircraft flying from Tokyo to Copenhagen with an interim stop at Anchorage developed gastrointestinal illness. The onset occurred shortly before the plane landed in Copenhagen after an 8½ hr flight from Anchorage. Epidemiologic investigation indicated that the food served to the passengers was prepared in Anchorage by a catering company owned by the airline. The item of food determined to be responsible for the outbreak was ham that had been handled by a cook who had an inflamed finger lesion from which *Staphylococcus aureus* was cultured. The ham had been held at room temperature for a sufficient length of time to allow the production of staphylococcal enterotoxin. Fortunately, except for 1 crew member who ate ham, none of the crew aboard the aircraft, including the pilots, became ill. Since it was suppertime for the crew, who had boarded the plane at Anchorage, they had been served a steak dinner instead of the breakfast meal at which the ham was served.

Food served aboard aircraft should be refrigerated prior to heating and serving. Food handlers on the ground and crew members who work in aircraft galleys should be educated in the proper handling techniques and particularly in the risk involved in storing foods at room temperature for prolonged periods.

This outbreak emphasizes the importance of serving pilots different food from that of the passengers and each other just before and during the flight.

Salmonellosis

Gastrointestinal illness was reported in 10 persons who had flown by commercial aircraft from Denver to Miami with an intermediate stop in Dallas on October 31, 1973. Stool specimens from 7 passengers on culture yielded *Salmonella thompson*. The breakfast meal served aboard the flight was implicated, although it was not possible to determine the specific item of food responsible for the outbreak.

Giardia lamblia Infection in Travellers to the Soviet Union

In July 1973, the Communicable Disease Center was notified of 3 cases of giardiasis in nurses who had returned from a tour of the Soviet Union. The nurses were members of one of three professional seminar tours sponsored by the American Association of Nurses-Anesthetists. There was a total of 399 tour participants. Information obtained from 80% of them revealed that 70 were diagnosed as having giardiasis on their return. Thirty had positive stool examinations. All members of the tour groups visited both Moscow and Leningrad. Infection was not related to the ingestion of uncooked vegetables or ice cream or eating at a specific restaurant. However, a history of drinking tap water was more common among cases than noncases.

Since 1963, a number of reports of infection with *Giardia lamblia* among travellers to the Soviet Union have been reported. Giardiasis should be considered in any person with a diarrheal illness lasting 1 week or longer who has recently traveled outside the United States. There is no known chemoprophylaxis for giardiasis. Measures such as avoiding ingestion of tap water and of uncooked, unpeeled fruits and vegetables may be effective in preventing giardiasis.

REFERENCES

CENT. DIS. CONTROL. 1974. Foodborne and waterborne disease outbreaks, 1973. U.S. Dep. Health, Educ. Welfare, Public Health Serv. Publ. (CDC) 75-8185.

CENT. DIS. CONTROL. 1975. Foodborne and waterborne disease outbreaks, 1974. U.S. Dep. Health, Educ. Welfare, Public Health Serv. Publ. (CDC) 76-8185.

CENT. DIS. CONTROL. 1976. Foodborne and waterborne disease outbreaks, 1975. U.S. Dep. Health, Educ. Welfare, Public Health Serv. Publ. (CDC) 77-8185.

CENT. DIS. CONTROL. 1977. Foodborne and waterborne disease outbreaks, 1976. U.S. Dep. Health, Educ. Welfare, Public Health Serv. Publ. (CDC) 78-8185.

COMMUNICABLE DIS. CENT. 1976. Diarrheal illness on a cruise ship by enterotoxic *Escherichia coli.* Morbidity Mortality *25,* 229.

FIUMARA, N. 1973. Giardiasis in travelers to the Soviet Union. N. Engl. J. Med. *288,* 1810.

U.S. DEP. HEALTH, EDUC. WELFARE. 1974. Salmonellosis on a Caribbean cruise ship. Morbidity Mortality Weekly Rep. *23* (39) 333.

U.S. DEP. HEALTH, EDUC. WELFARE. 1975. Outbreak of staphylococcal food poisoning aboard an aircraft. Morbidity Mortality Weekly Rep. *24* (7) 57.

U.S. DEP. HEALTH, EDUC. WELFARE. 1976. Diarrheal illness on a cruise ship caused by enterotoxigenic *Escherichia coli.* Morbidity Mortality Weekly Rep. *25* (29) 229.

U.S. DEP. HEALTH, EDUC. WELFARE, PUBLIC HEALTH SERV. 1974. Survey of the incidence of gastrointestinal illness in cruise ship passengers. Morbidity Mortality Weekly Rep. *23,* 65.

WALZER, P.D., WOLFE, M.S. and SCHULTZ, M.G. 1970. Giardiasis in travelers. J. Infect. Dis. *124,* 235.

28

Statistical Report of Foodborne and Waterborne Disease Outbreaks

The information following is taken from the latest available Summary of Foodborne and Waterborne Disease Outbreaks reported in 1977 to the Center for Disease Control, Bureau of Epidemiology, U.S. Public Health Service, and was issued in August 1979 (Cent. Dis. Control 1979).

FOODBORNE DISEASE OUTBREAKS

Consumers, physicians, hospital personnel, and persons involved with food service or food processing report on complaints of illness believed to be caused by food to health departments or other regulatory agencies. Local health department personnel (epidemiologists, sanitarians, public health nurses, etc.) carry out most epidemiologic investigations of these reports and make their findings available, through channels, to the Center for Disease Control (CDC). The two federal regulatory agencies which have major responsibilities for food protection, the Food and Drug Administration (FDA) and the Department of Agriculture (USDA), report episodes of foodborne illness to the CDC and to state and local health authorities which, in turn, report to FDA and USDA any foodborne disease outbreaks that might involve commercial products. If an outbreak is extensive or involves products that move in interstate commerce, the CDC will participate in the investigation on special request. In addition, CDC is alerted to the possible occurrence of botulism by pharmaceutical manufacturers who report to the center all requests for botulinal antitoxin.

During 1977 there were 436 outbreaks of foodborne disease involving 9896 cases reported in the United States. The etiology of the outbreaks was confirmed in 157 instances in which illness occurred in 4072 persons. Bacterial contamination was found to be responsible for 101 of the outbreaks resulting in 3454 cases. Chemicals caused 37 outbreaks with 455 cases, parasites were incriminated in 15 outbreaks with 91 cases, and viruses were involved in 4 outbreaks with 72 cases (Table 28.1).

TABLE 28.1. FOODBORNE DISEASE OUTBREAKS WITH CONFIRMED ETIOLOGY RE-
PORTED TO U.S. PUBLIC HEALTH SERVICE, 1977

Etiology	Outbreaks	Cases
Bacterial		
Arizona hinshawii	1	13
Clostridium botulinum	20	75
C. perfringens	6	568
Salmonella	41	1706
Shigella	5	67
Staphylococcus	25	905
Vibrio cholerae	1	2
V. parahaemolyticus	2	118
Total	101	3454
Chemical		
Heavy metal	8	326
Fish poisoning (ciguatoxin		
and scombrotoxin)	16	93
Monosodium glutamate	2	11
Mushroom poisoning	5	14
Other chemicals	6	11
Total	37	455
Parasites		
Trichinella spiralis	14	87
Anisakidae	1	4
Total	15	91
Viral		
Hepatitis	4	72
Total	4	72
CONFIRMED TOTAL	157	4072

Source: Cent. Dis. Control, Public Health Serv. (1977).

The report from the CDC can not be considered to give the absolute
incidence of the outbreaks of foodborne diseases of various etiologies that
have occurred during the year. For example, diseases with short incubation periods, such as in outbreaks caused by staphylococci or in chemical poisoning, are more likely to be recognized as common source foodborne disease outbreaks and reported to health authorities. On the other
hand, diseases with an incubation period of several weeks, such as hepatitis, are likely to escape detection as a common source infection and fail to
be reported as such. Outbreaks of serious diseases, such as botulism or
mushroom poisoning, are more likely to be reported than less serious
illnesses, but because of their rarity are apt not to be recognized and
diagnosed. Outbreaks of *Clostridium perfringens* are recognized readily
but are rarely confirmed because specimens have to be adequately transported and cultured under anaerobic conditions. Outbreaks of *Bacillus
cereus, Escherichia coli, Vibrio parahaemolyticus*, and *Yersinia enterocolitica* are probably less likely to be confirmed as these organisms are
less often considered clinically, epidemiologically, and in the laboratory.
In outbreaks of unknown etiology, the accuracy of reported information
is always suspect.

Eight deaths were associated with foodborne outbreaks. Five deaths were attributed to eating food containing the toxin of *Clostridium botulinum*. The other 3 deaths occurred in persons who consumed herbal teas. The reliability of these figures is also questionable as many deaths are not immediate and in a number of the reports it was not indicated whether or not death occurred. When death is not immediate, foodborne disease may not be appreciated as contributing to the demise of an elderly or debilitated person unable to withstand otherwise minor physical stresses.

One should understand the limitation of the quantity and quality of the data in the CDC report as it obviously represents merely a fraction of the actual number of outbreaks and cases of foodborne diseases that occurred during the year.

In spite of its deficiencies, much may be learned from the information contained in the report. For example, it enumerates the food items that were responsible for the reported outbreaks; it indicates the types of places where the incriminated foods were eaten; and it specifies the establishments where mishandling of the foods took place.

The vehicles of transmission were identified in 267 (61%) of the outbreaks; multiple vehicles were involved in 19 (6.7%). Of the 338 outbreaks in which a single vehicle was identified, meats or poultry were incriminated in 74 (31%), Oriental food in 32 (12%), salads including chicken, turkey, potato, and egg in 12 (5%), fish or shellfish in 31 (12%), dairy products in 7 (3%), fruits and vegetables in 8 (3%), mushrooms in 5 (2%), and other foods in 23 (9%). Of the meat vehicles, beef, ham, and sausage were most frequently incriminated.

Outbreaks of botulism frequently involved home preserved vegetables. *C. perfringens* was usually transmitted by beef, and staphylococcal infections most often involved meat. Salmonellae outbreaks were caused by many different vehicles, including meat, such as processed roast beef, poultry, dairy products, and salads. The outbreaks of heavy metal poisoning all involved nondairy beverages stored in metal containers or in contact with tubing of a type that allowed metallic ions to dissolve in the beverage. Fish poisoning was caused by coral reef fish (groupers). Trichinosis outbreaks involved pork or sausage.

In three-quarters of the outbreaks, the food was eaten at home (25%) or in a restaurant (48%). Of the 20 outbreaks of botulism, the food was consumed at home in 16 (80%), in a restaurant once (5%), and was unknown in 3 (15%). Chemical outbreaks occurred frequently in the home and in food service establishments. Outbreaks caused by parasites usually occurred at home, while the hepatitis outbreaks resulted from food eaten at food service establishments.

The places where mishandling of the food resulted in illness were given in 393 outbreaks. Of these, food service establishments (such as restaurants, cafeterias, hospitals, industrial plants) were specified as being responsible for the mishandling in 73%, homes in 25%, and food-processing establishments where food is prepared for marketing in 2%.

The majority of outbreaks of *C. perfringens*, salmonellae, and staphylococci were traced to food service establishments, while most of the cases of trichinosis occurred in the home.

The implication of a food-processing establishment's mishandling food is great both to the public health and to the establishment concerned. Consequently the outbreaks attributed to these establishments are thoroughly investigated and reported data are carefully scrutinized. For these reasons such data are considered highly reliable. Reports have indicated that 8 outbreaks causing 342 cases were attributed to mishandling of food in food-processing establishments in 1977. During 1976, these establishments were responsible for 15 outbreaks with 1283 cases (see Table 28.2).

TABLE 28.2. FOODBORNE DISEASE OUTBREAKS CAUSED BY MISHANDLING IN FOOD-PROCESSING ESTABLISHMENTS, 1976 AND 1977

Etiology	Vehicle	Number of Cases
Outbreaks in 1976		
Salmonella heidelberg	Cheese	339
S. bovis-morbificans	Precooked roast beef	21
S. infantis	Nutrient supplement	4
Staphylococcus Enterotoxin D	Greek spaghetti	20
Staphylococcus	Beef ravioli	4
Staphylococcus Enterotoxin D	Custard-filled doughnuts	2
Staphylococcus	Pepperoni, sausage	3
Yersinia enterocolitica	Chocolate milk	286
Sodium nitrate	Table salt	2
Propyl paraben	Cake icing	9
Histamine	Cheese	38
Niacin	Hamburger	2
Niacin	Cubed steak	3
Unknown	Tuna extender	508
Unknown	Milk	42
Total: 15 outbreaks		1283
Outbreaks in 1977		
Salmonella infantis	Barbecued pork	17
S. newport	Precooked roast beef	100
S. typhimurium	Cake icing	3
S. typhimurium	Precooked roast beef	8
Staphylococcus Enterotoxin	Whipped butter	200
Senecio longilobus	Herbal tea	1
Fish poisoning (2 outbreaks)	Tuna	13
Total: 8 outbreaks		342

Source: Cent. Dis. Control, Public Health Serv. (1977).

The 1977 data reflected patterns of disease causation seen in previous years. In reported outbreaks of botulism and trichinosis, the most frequent error was inadequate cooking of the food. Improper holding temperature most frequently contributed to reported outbreaks of *C. per-fringens*, salmonellae, and staphylococci intoxication. Improper storage of beverages in metal receptacles or tubing was the most important contributing factor in the outbreaks of heavy metal poisoning. In other chemical poisonings, the food was obtained from an unsafe source. In the 4 outbreaks of hepatitis, a person suspected of having active hepatitis was involved in food handling. In the outbreaks of mushroom and fish poisoning, the food was originally unsafe.

Generally, outbreaks were distributed more or less equally throughout the year. Outbreaks caused by salmonellae and staphylococci tended to occur more frequently in the summer months, probably because the warm temperatures allow bacteria to grow in unrefrigerated foods.

WATERBORNE DISEASE OUTBREAKS

Waterborne disease outbreaks, like foodborne outbreaks, are reported to the CDC by state health departments. In addition, the Health Effects Research Laboratory, Environmental Protection Agency (EPA), contacts all state water supply agencies in order to obtain information about waterborne disease outbreaks and assists local and state health departments in their epidemiologic investigations. The CDC and EPA also offer expert recommendations in the engineering and environmental aspects of water purification, and, when indicated, provide large volume water sampling for the isolation and identification of viruses, parasites, and specific bacterial pathogens.

Municipal water systems are defined as public or investor-owned water supplies that serve large or small communities, subdivisions, and trailer parks of at least 15 service connections or 25 year-round residents. Semipublic water systems are present systems in institutions, industries, camps, parks, hotels, and service stations which have their own water system available for use by the general public. Individual water systems, generally wells and springs, are those used by single or several residents or by persons travelling outside of populated areas (e.g., backpackers).

Data of waterborne disease outbreaks included in the CDC summary have limitations similar to those mentioned in the foodborne disease section of the summary. It must likewise be interpreted with caution since it represents only a small part of a large public health problem. The data, however, are helpful in revealing the various etiologies of waterborne diseases, the seasonal occurrence of outbreaks, the types of systems most vulnerable, and the deficiencies in the systems that most frequently result in outbreaks.

Table 28.3 shows the number of outbreaks and cases by etiology and type of water system. Of 34 outbreaks, 20 (59%) were designated as

TABLE 28.3. WATERBORNE DISEASE OUTBREAKS BY ETIOLOGY AND TYPE OF WATER SYSTEM, 1977

	Municipal		Semipublic		Individual		Total	
	Outbreaks	Cases	Outbreaks	Cases	Outbreaks	Cases	Outbreaks	Cases
Acute gastro-intestinal illness	5	518	13	1396	2	24	20	1938
Chemical poisoning	4	612	1	11	1	10	6	633
Giardiasis	2	950	2	62	0	0	4	1012
Salmonellosis	1	206	1	7	0	0	2	213
Hepatitis	0	0	1	47	0	0	1	47
Shigellosis	0	0	1	17	0	0	1	17
Total	12	2286	19	1540	3	34	34	3860

Source: Cent. Dis. Control, Public Health Serv. (1977).

"acute gastrointestinal illness." This category includes outbreaks characterized by upper and/or lower gastrointestinal symptomatology for which no special etiologic agent was identified. There were 14 (41%) outbreaks of known etiology: chemical 6, *Giardia lamblia* 4, salmonellae 2, *Shigella* 1, and hepatitis 1. In 3 of the 5 largest outbreaks, an etiologic agent was found: *Giardia lamblia* in a municipal water system in New Hampshire (750 cases), photographic developer fluid (hydroquinone) aboard a U.S. Navy vessel in California (531 cases), and *Salmonella typhimurium* in a municipal water system in Iowa (206 cases). There were 3 outbreaks caused by contaminated ice, and 1 outbreak in which contaminated water was used to make whipped cream.

It is important that an attempt be made to isolate pathogens from the water supply during an outbreak to help establish the etiology, but it is equally important to also determine the presence of coliforms and document their relative importance as indicator organisms for use in routine surveillance of water supplies.

Attention is called to the fact that the absence of coliform bacilli in a water supply does not necessarily indicate that it is free from fecal contamination, as regular chlorination may eliminate the coliforms but has no effect on *Giardia* cysts or *Entamoeba histolytica* cysts, both of them requiring a high concentration of chlorine and a longer contact time for their inactivation. Of the 6 chemical outbreaks, 3 were due to toxic amounts of copper leaching from plumbing due to corrosive water and a low pH. The other water contaminants were fluoride, gasoline, and photographic developer.

Most outbreaks involved semipublic (56%) and municipal (35%) water systems, and fewer involved individual (9%) systems. Outbreaks attributed to water from municipal systems affected an average of 191 persons compared with 81 persons in outbreaks involving semipublic systems and 11 persons in outbreaks associated with individual water systems. Deficiencies in treatment (inadequately or untreated water) accounted for 26 (76%) of the outbreaks. Untreated water (surface or ground) accounted for 14 of these 26 outbreaks (Table 28.4). Of the 19 outbreaks associated with semipublic water supply systems, 15 (79%) involved visitors to areas mostly for recreational purposes, 13 outbreaks occurring in the summer months, May through September.

TABLE 28.4. WATERBORNE DISEASE OUTBREAKS BY TYPE OF SYSTEM, AND CAUSE OF SYSTEM DEFICIENCY, 1977

	Municipal		Semipublic		Individual		Total	
	Outbreaks	Cases	Outbreaks	Cases	Outbreaks	Cases	Outbreaks	Cases
Untreated surface water	1	200	1	55	1	12	3	267
Untreated groundwater	0	0	9	547	2	22	11	569
Treatment deficiencies	4	1362	8	891	0	0	12	2253
Deficiencies in distribution system	6	718	1	47	0	0	7	765
Miscellaneous	1	0	0	0	0	0	1	6
Total	12	2286	19	1540	3	34	34	3860

Source: Cent. Dis. Control, Public Health Serv. (1977).

This indicates that semipublic water systems in national, state, and local parks must be routinely reappraised and monitored with corrections made to ensure safe water under increased demands by large numbers of visitors. The large outbreaks that occurred in 1975 in Crater Lake National Park with more than 1000 cases, and in 1977 in Yellowstone National Park with more than 400 cases, underscore the actual and potential problems that occur in recreational areas.

The outbreak of hepatitis occurred after an unknown cross-connecting pipe was accidentally broken during the repair of a septic tank inflow line. Sewage discharging from the septic tank line entered the broken piping that connected directly to a nearby (46 m or 50 yd) unchlorinated groundwater well which had previously provided safe drinking water. This outbreak illustrates the hazards of contaminating an established safe source during nearby repair work involving pipes and sewerage lines. During such repairs, unchlorinated drinking supplies should be temporarily chlorinated and such water should be closely monitored bacteriologically during and for some time after the repair work is completed to ensure its potability.

REFERENCES

BRYAN, F.L. 1972. Emerging foodborne diseases surveillance and epidemiology. Factors that contribute to outbreaks and their control. J. Milk Food Technol. *35*, 618.

CENT. DIS. CONTROL. 1979. Foodborne and Waterborne Disease Surveillance, Annual Summary, 1977. Cent. Dis. Control, Bur. Epidemiol., U.S. Public Health Serv., Dep. Health, Educ. Welfare, Atlanta.

CENT. DIS. CONTROL, PUBLIC HEALTH SERV. 1977. Foodborne and waterborne disease outbreaks. U.S. Dep. Health, Educ. Welfare, Public Health Serv. Publ. (CDC) 78−8185.

CRAUN, G.F. and McCABE, L.J. 1973. Review of the causes of waterborne disease outbreaks. J. Am. Water Works Assoc. 65, 74.

KIMM, V.J. and ANGELETTI, R. 1977. Who safeguards your drinking water? Prof. Nutr. 9 (1) 1.

Glossary

In order to familiarize the reader with the technical terms and medical terminology that appear in the text, the following glossary is presented.

Abattoir Slaughterhouse.

Acidosis A condition in which there is an excess of acid products in the blood or excreted in the urine; when the condition gives rise to morbid symptoms, it is called **acid intoxication**.

Adenopathy Swelling of and morbid changes in the lymph nodes.

Agglutination test A test in which there is a loss of motility and aggregation in small masses of microorganisms in a culture when a specific immune serum is added.

Ameba A unicellular protozoan organism; some may be parasitic and pathogenic.

Anaerobic organism One that lives and grows in the absence of oxygen.

Anorexia Loss of appetite.

Antibody Any substance in the bloodstream or other fluids of the body which exerts a specific restrictive or destructive action on bacteria or other noxious products, or neutralizes their toxin; examples are antitoxins, precipitins, agglutinins, lysins, and immune bodies.

Antitoxin A substance in the serum which binds and neutralizes toxin.

Arachnida A class of arthropods comprised mostly of air-breathing invertebrates, including spiders, scorpions, mites, and ticks having 4 pairs of legs and no antennae.

Arthralgia Severe pain in a joint, especially when inflammation is involved.

Ascites An accumulation of serous fluid in the abdominal cavity.

Bacillus A genus of the class Schizomycetes of a generally rod-shaped or elongated form varying considerably in shape and size; they divide transversely and may be found in threads or chains.

Bacteremia The presence of living bacteria in the circulating blood.

Bacteriophage A lytic (destructive) agent assumed to be an ultra-microbe parasitic to ordinary microorganisms and causing their dissolution.

b.i.d. Abbreviation of Latin *bi in die*, twice a day.

Biopsy Examination of tissue excised from the human body.

Blepharoptosia Drooping of the upper eyelid.

Bubo An enlargement of a lymphatic gland, usually in the groin or axilla, often going on to suppurative inflammation.

Cardiovascular Relating to the heart and blood vessels or the circulation.

Carrier An infected person or animal that harbors a specific infectious agent in the absence of clinical disease and serves as a potential source of infection for man.

Casiation A form of degeneration in which tissues are transformed into a cheesy mass resembling pus thickened in consistency.

Cellulitis Inflammation of cellular or connective tissue.

Cercaria The final larval stage of the trematode worms; it consists of a body and elongated tail resembling a tadpole and is free swimming.

Cestode A tapeworm.

Chlorination The addition of chlorine in the treatment of a water supply.

Cholecystitis Inflammation of the gallbladder.

Cirrhosis A degeneration of the parenchyma cells of an organ such as the liver, with hypertrophy of the interstitial connective tissue.

Colon The portion of the large intestine extending from the cecum to the rectum.

Contact A person or animal that has been in close association with an infected person or a contaminated environment.

Convalescence The time elapsing between the termination of a disease and the patient's complete restoration to health.

Cysticercus The encysted larva of various tapeworms.

Dehydration The losing of water.

Disinfection The destruction of infectious agents outside the body by chemical or physical means.

Diplopia Double vision due to paralysis of the ocular muscles in consequence of which the image of an object falls upon noncorresponding portions of the 2 retinas.

Edema An abnormal accumulation of clear watery fluid in the lymph spaces of the tissues (dropsy).

Electrolyte A compound when dissolved in water contains ions such as sodium or potassium required by the body.

Empyema An accumulation of pus in the pleural cavity.

Encephalitis Inflammation of the brain.

Endemic Referring to a disease peculiar to a locality or region.

Endocarditis Inflammation of the lining membrane within the heart.

Enteric Pertaining to the intestine.

Enterotoxin A toxin that is specific for the cells of the mucous membrane of the intestine.

Enzyme An organic substance secreted by the body cells which acts as a ferment inducing chemical changes in other substances by catalysis, itself remaining apparently unchanged in the process.

Eosinophilia An increase in the number of eosinophils in the blood.

Epidemic The occurrence in a community or region of cases of an illness clearly in excess of normal expectancy and derived from a common or a propagated source.

Epidemiology The science that deals with the incidence, distribution, clinical nature, reservoir of infection, mode of transmission, laboratory diagnosis, and methods of control and prevention of disease in a population; the epidemiologist is sometimes referred to as a "disease detective."

Epistaxis Nosebleed.

Etiologic agent An agent, chemical, physical, or biological, responsible for producing an effect, such as an illness.

Exanthem A skin eruption occurring as a symptom of a general disease.

Flatulence The presence of an excessive amount of gas in the stomach and intestine.

Fomite An inanimate object not supporting bacterial growth but capable of transmitting pathogenic microorganisms from a sick person to a susceptible host.

Food infection A condition in which a pathogenic enteric microorganism enters the gastrointestinal tract in contaminated food, multiplies, and attacks the intestinal tissues, causing illness.

Food poisoning A condition in which a chemical agent, or a poisonous plant or animal, or a bacterial toxin present in food before it is eaten causes an intoxication when it is consumed.

Gastralgia Stomachache.

Gastrointestinal Pertaining to the stomach and the intestine.

Gingivitis Inflammation of the gums.

Glomerulonephritis A form of nephritis (inflammation of the kidneys) with pronounced lesions of the glomeruli (the plexus of capillaries).

Granuloma A circumscribed collection of epithelioid cells and leucocytes resembling granulation tissue (as on the surface of a healing wound) surrounding a central point of irritation.

Halophilic The ability to flourish in a salty environment.

Helminth An intestinal worm parasite.

Hematuria The passage of blood in the urine.

Hemolysis Destruction of the erythrocytes (red blood cells).

Hemoptysis Bleeding from the lungs or bronchial tubes.

Host A living organism (man or animal) on which a parasite lives.

Hypokalemia Deficiency of potassium in the blood.

Icteric Marked by jaundice.

Immune person An individual who possesses specific antibodies or cellular immunity to a disease because of previous infection or artificial immunization; or a natural state in which the body is resistant to a specific disease.

Immunization
  (1) **Active immunization** The administration of a vaccine in order to artificially produce a lasting protection against a specific disease.
  (2) **Passive immunization** The administration of an antitoxin or immune serum to temporarily protect a person who has been exposed to a specific disease.

Incubation period The time interval between the exposure to an infectious disease, or the ingestion of a contaminated food or a noxious product, and the appearance of the first sign or symptom of illness.

Infectious agent A microorganism or other parasitic organism capable of producing infection or infectious disease.

Insecticide A chemical substance capable of destroying arthropods (insects).

Keratoconjunctivitis Inflammation of the cornea and conjunctiva.

Larva The immature form of an insect or worm on issuing from the egg.

Lymphadenopathy Disease of the lymph glands.

Lymphadenitis Inflammation of lymph nodes.

Melena The passage of dark colored tarry stools due to the presence of blood altered by the intestinal juices.

Meningitis Inflammation of the membranes of the brain or spinal cord.

Methemoglobinemia The presence of methemoglobin (transformed oxyhemoglobin) in the blood.

Miracidium The embryo of the fluke.

Mydriasis Dilatation of the pupil.

Myocarditis Inflammation of the muscular wall of the heart.

Necrosis The local death of more or less extensive groups of cells with degenerative changes.

Nematode Round or thread-like parasitic worm.

Neurotoxin A toxin that attacks nerve tissue.

Night soil Human excrement collected for fertilizing the soil.

Ophthalmitis Inflammation of the structures of the eye.

Osteomyelitis Inflammation of the bone marrow.

Otitis media Inflammation of the middle ear.

Parasite An animal or vegetable organism that lives on or in another and draws its nourishment therefrom.

Parenteral In some way other than by the intestinal canal; referring to the introduction of medicinal material into the veins or subcutaneous tissues.

Paresthesia An abnormal spontaneous sensation such as of burning, pricking, or numbness.

Pasteurization The terms "pasteurization," "pasteurized," and similar terms shall mean the process of heating every particle of milk or milk product to at least 62.8°C (145°F), and holding it continuously at or above this temperature for at least 30 min; or to at least 71.7°C (161°F), and holding it continuously at or above this temperature for at least 15 sec; in equipment which is properly operated and approved by the health authority; provided that: milk products which have a higher milkfat content than milk and/or contain added sweeteners shall be heated to at least 65.6°C (150°F), and held continuously at or above this temperature for at least 30 min; or to at least 74.4°C (166°F), and held continuously at or above this temperature for at least 15 sec; provided further that: nothing in this definition shall be construed as barring any other pasteurization process which has been recognized by the United States Public Health Service to be equally efficient and which is approved by the state health authority.

Pathogenic Capable of causing disease in a susceptible host.

Pericarditis Inflammation of the membrane enclosing the heart.

Peritonitis Inflammation of the serous membrane lining the abdominal wall and enveloping the contained viscera.

Peritonsillar abscess An abscess in the tissues around the tonsil.

Petechia Minute hemorrhagic spot of pinpoint to pinhead size in the skin.

Peyer's patches Aggregated glands; collections of many lymphoid nodules closely packed together and forming oblong elevations of the mucous membrane of the small intestine.

Pharyngitis Inflammation of the mucous membrane and underlying parts of the pharynx.

Placentitis Inflammation of the placenta.

Pneumonitis Inflammation of the lungs.

Prophylaxis The prevention of disease.

Prostration A marked loss of strength; exhaustion.

Protozoa A phylum of the animal kingdom made up of organisms consisting of a single cell.

Ptomaine poisoning A meaningless term formerly used to indicate food poisoning or infection; it is derived from *ptoma* meaning corpse and is no longer used.

Purgative A cathartic.

Pyelonephritis Inflammation of the kidney with special involvement of the renal pelvis.

Refrigeration (Pertaining to perishable foods) Storage of foods at low temperature (4.4° to 7.2°C or 40° to 45°F).

Regurgitation The act of vomiting; to expel the contents of the stomach.

Reservoir of infection A human being, animal, arthropod, plant, or soil in which an infective agent lives and multiplies and can be transmitted to a susceptible host.

Salivation Excessive secretion of saliva.

Sanitation The employment of measures designed to promote health and prevent disease through personal hygiene, physical, chemical, and microbial cleanliness of food, and proper environmental control.

Scatological Related to excrement.

Scolex The head of a tapeworm by which it is attached to the wall of the intestine.

Septicemia A systemic disease caused by the presence of microorganisms or their toxins in the circulating blood.

Serotype The type of microorganism determined by its constituent antigens.

Splenomegaly Enlargement of the spleen.

Spondylitis Inflammation of vertebrae.

Spore A reproductive cell of a protozoan or a lower plant.

Tenesmus Ineffective effort at defecation.

Teratogenic The development of an abnormality in the fetus.

Thermolabile Unstable when heated; destroyed by heat.

Thermostable Stable when heated; retaining its characteristic properties on being moderately heated.

t.i.d. Abbreviation of Latin *ter in die*, 3 times a day.

Toxin A poisonous substance elaborated during the growth of certain pathogenic microorganisms.

Tracheotomy Incision of the trachea especially for the insertion of a tube to facilitate breathing.

Trematodes Any of the parasitic flatworms, including the flukes.

Trophozoite The active motile feeding stage of a protozoan organism as contrasted with the nonmotile encysted stage.

Ubiquity Presence everywhere or in many places simultaneously.

Vaccination The act of administering a vaccine for the prevention of a disease.

Vector A term noting an insect that transports a pathogenic microorganism from the sick to the well, either (1) by soiling its feet or proboscis, (2) by passing the organism through its gastrointestinal tract, or (3) through its bite.

V_i phage tests *Salmonella typhi* can be differentiated into several types by means of bacteriophage (phage) typing. Bacteriophage is an ultra microscopic agent, a form of bacterial virus, that under appropriate conditions multiplies in the presence of bacteria and causes their dissolution. There are a number of recognized phage types of *S. typhi*.

A certain strain of bacteriophage propagates in the presence of a given strain of *S. typhi* and becomes specific for that strain. By virtue of their specificity, phages are useful in epidemiologic work. Phage typing aids in tracing the origin of infection of a case or an outbreak of typhoid fever.

Index

hogs, 154
humans, 154
Taenia solium, 153
central nervous system, 153
eyes, 153
heart, 153
striated muscle, 153
subcutaneous tissues, 153
treatment, 155
oleoresin of aspidium, 155
quinacrine hydrochloride, 155

Daffodils, 196
Daphne, 197, 202
Daphne mezereon, 206
DDT, DDE, DDD, 174
Deerfly fever, 92
Delaney Amendment, 181
Dermacentor andersoni, 93
Dermacentor variabolis, 93
Dieffenbachia, 196, 198
"dumb cane," 196, 198
Diethylpyrocarbonate (DEP), 181
Diethylstilbestrol (DES), 181
Diodoquin, 134
Diphtheria, 107–108
carriers, 108
procaine penicillin, 108
case fatality, 107
contacts, 107–108
cultures, 108
toxoid boosters, 108
Corynebacterium diphtheriae, 107
disinfection, 107
epidemics, 108
immunization, 107
incubation period, 107
isolation of patient, 107
laboratory examination, 107
nose and throat cultures, 107
quarantine of contacts, 107
restriction of food handlers, 107
toxin, 107
myocarditis, 107
nerve paralysis, 107
suffocation, 107
toxoid, 107
transmission, 107
treatment, 108
antibiotics, 108
antitoxin, 108
Diphyllobothriasis, 156–157
broad tapeworm, 156
control, 157

adequate sewerage, 157
education, 157
freezing of fish, 157
handwashing, 157
sanitary measures, 157
thorough cooking of fish, 157
diagnosis, 157
eggs in feces, 157
Diphyllobothrium latum, 156
fish tapeworm, 156
life cycle, 156
symptoms, 157
transmission, 156
raw freshwater fish, 156
treatment, 157
(as in taeniasis), 155
Diphyllobothrium latum, 156
Dog tapeworm disease, 137, 155
Dogfish, 214
Dulcin, 181
Dwarf tapeworm disease, 137, 157–158
Dysentery, 35. *See also* Shigellosis and
Amebiasis

Echinococcus, 155
E. granulosus, 155
E. multilocularis, 155–156
Eel, 214
Embargo suspected food, 54
Emetine hydrochloride, 161
Emulsifiers, 180
Endrin, 174
Entamoeba histolytica, 127, 129–130, 136
Enterobiasis, 147–150
diagnosis, 147
presence of worms, 147
Scotch® cellulose adhesive tape sampling, 148–149
Enterobius vermicularis, 147–148, 150
life cycle, 147
oxyuriasis, 147–150
pinworm disease, 147–150
prevention of spread, 148–149
symptoms, 147
anal itching, 147
anorexia, 147
diarrhea, 147
irritability, 147
secondary infections, 147
treatment, 150
Piperazine citrate, 150
Pyrvinium pamoate, 150
Enterotoxin, 2
Enzymes, 180

rodents, 124
symptoms, 124
Hemorrhagic jaundice, 97
Hepatic capillariasis, 137, 152–153, *See also* Intestinal capillariasis
Capillaria hepatica, 153
  diagnosis, 153
  eosinophilia, 153
  life cycle, 153
  prevention, 153
    prevent food contamination with soil,
      153
    protection of water supply, 153
  reservoir of infection, 152
    rat, 152
  symptoms, 153
    ascites, 153
    hepatitis, 153
    weight loss, 153
Hepatitis, 111–122
  viral, 2, 111, 266–267, 270–271
Hexylresorcinol, 145, 159
Home canning, 50, 52, 54, 267
Hormones, 176
  banned by FDA, 176
    carcinogenic, 176
    to promote growth in beef, 176
  diethylstilbestrol (DES), 176
    female sex hormone, 176
Houseplants, 196–198
Hyacinths, 196
Hydatidosis, 135, 137, 155–156
  control, 156
    dogs' feces disposal, 155
  dog tapeworm, 155
  Echinococcus granulosus, 155
    infective eggs, 155
    life cycle, 155
    symptoms, 155–156
    transmission, 155
      contaminated food and water, 155
      hand-to-mouth transfer, 155
    unilocular echinococcosis, 155
  Echinococcus multilocularis, 155–156
    alveolar hydatid disease, 156
    diagnosis, 156
      microscopic examination, 156
        feces, 156
        ruptured cyst, 156
        sputum, 156
        urine, 156
    hand-to-mouth spread, 156
  reservoir of infection, 155
    dingoes, 155
    dogs, 155
    foxes, 155–156
    wolves, 155–156

Hymenolepiasis, 137, 157–158
  dwarf tapeworm disease, 157
  Hymenolepis nana, 157
  incubation period, 158
  ova in feces, 158
  prevention, 158
  reservoir of infection, 157–158
  symptoms, 158
  transmission, 158
    direct contact, 158
    food, 158
    hand-to-mouth spread, 158
  treatment, 158
    quinacrine hydrochloride, 158

Ichthyosarcotoxism, 214
Immunization, 4
Infectious hepatitis, 35, 111–123
  characteristics, 112
  control, 112
    isolation of patient, 112
    prophylactic gamma globulin, 112
    restricting sick food handlers, 112
    sanitary disposal of feces and urine, 112
  diagnosis, 113
    liver function tests, 113
  epidemics, 111–121
  fatality rate, 112
  hepatitis, 111
    viral type, 111
    Virus A, 111
    Virus B, 111
  incubation period, 112
  investigation of outbreaks, 113
    Elmont outbreak, 114–121
  prevention, 112
    avoid questionable raw shellfish, 112
    gamma globulin to contacts, 112
    personal hygiene, 112
    proper sanitation, 112
    protection of water supply, 112
    reporting, 112
    sanitary sewage disposal, 112
    use of sterile needles and syringes, 112
  sources of infection, 111
  symptoms, 112
  transmission, 111
    fecal-oral route, 112
    orally, 111
    parenterally, 111
  treatment, 113
    antihistamines, 113
    diet, 113
    intravenous glucose, 113

Other AVI Books

BASIC FOOD MICROBIOLOGY
Banwart
CLINICAL MICROBIOLOGY
DiLiello
ELEMENTARY FOOD SCIENCE
2nd Edition   *Nickerson and Ronsivalli*
EVALUATION OF PROTEINS FOR HUMANS
Bodwell
FOOD AND BEVERAGE MYCOLOGY
Beuchat
FOOD MICROBIOLOGY: PUBLIC HEALTH AND SPOILAGE
ASPECTS
deFigueiredo and Splittstoesser
FOOD PROCESSING WASTE MANAGEMENT
Green and Kramer
FOOD QUALITY ASSURANCE
Gould
FOOD SANITATION
Guthrie
FOOD SERVICE SCIENCE
Smith and Minor
FUNCTIONAL MEDICAL LABORATORY TECHNOLOGY   *Rothstein*
Clinical Bacteriology   *Scimone*
Clinical Chemistry   *Scimone and Rothstein*
Hematology and Urinalysis   *Lamberg and Rothstein*
Histology and Cytology   *Lamberg and Rothstein*
Serology, Immunology & Blood Banking   *Williams*
FUNDAMENTALS OF FOOD MICROBIOLOGY
Fields
IMMUNOLOGICAL ASPECTS OF FOOD
Catsimpoolas
LABORATORY MANUAL IN FOOD CHEMISTRY
Woods and Aurand
PRINCIPLES OF FOOD PACKAGING
2nd Edition   *Sacharow and Griffin*
PROCESSED MEATS
Kramlich, Pearson and Tauber
SCHOOL FOODSERVICE
Van Egmond
THE FREEZING PRESERVATION OF FOODS   4th Edition
Vol. 1, 2, 3 and 4   *Tressler, Van Arsdel and Copley*
THE SAFETY OF FOODS
2nd Edition   *Graham*